Before We Teach Music

Before We Teach Music

The Resonant Legacies of Childhoods and Children

LORI A. CUSTODERO

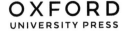

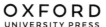

Oxford University Press is a department of the University of Oxford. It furthers
the University's objective of excellence in research, scholarship, and education
by publishing worldwide. Oxford is a registered trade mark of Oxford University
Press in the UK and certain other countries.

Published in the United States of America by Oxford University Press
198 Madison Avenue, New York, NY 10016, United States of America.

© Oxford University Press 2024

All rights reserved. No part of this publication may be reproduced, stored in
a retrieval system, or transmitted, in any form or by any means, without the
prior permission in writing of Oxford University Press, or as expressly permitted
by law, by license, or under terms agreed with the appropriate reproduction
rights organization. Inquiries concerning reproduction outside the scope of the
above should be sent to the Rights Department, Oxford University Press, at the
address above.

You must not circulate this work in any other form
and you must impose this same condition on any acquirer.

Library of Congress Control Number: 2023952607

ISBN 978-0-19-755788-4 (pbk.)
ISBN 978-0-19-755787-7 (hbk.)

DOI: 10.1093/oso/9780197557877.001.0001

Contents

Foreword	vii
1. Musical Beings	1
Childhood, Children, and Music	1
Living in Music: Experiences of Time and Movement	4
Feeling of Music: Expression, Communication, and Comfort	9
Before We Teach	14
2. "Prelude to a Method": Memories, Music, and Childhood	17
Introduction	17
Childhood and the Historical Self	18
Reconstructing and Remembering	21
Environments, Development, and Disposition	24
Kaleidoscopic Turns: Seeing through New Eyes	29
3. Forming Relationships: Music in Early Childhood	35
Accessing and Sharing Memories	35
Family as Sound Group: Music, Ritual, and Spontaneity	38
Music and Family Member Roles: Learning to Be Together	43
Music in Neighborhood and Societal Contexts	52
Constructing a Musical Self through Relationships	55
4. A Sense of Musical Self: Engaging Dispositions and Claiming Identities	61
Conceptualizing Musical Selves	61
Dispositions and the Power of Implicit Knowing	62
Dispositional Personality Traits and Motivating Conditions	67
Instrument Choice and Identity	75
Finding Musical Kin	78
A Sense of Musical Self	83
5. Musical Pathways: Disruption and Renewal in Musical Lives	87
Road Trips	87
Disruption and Renewal of Musical Plans	88
Clara (1999)	90
Jeremy (2016)	92
Ruth (2016)	98
Claudia (2010)	103
Teaching Narratives and Generativity	107

6. Encounters with Children: Lessons on Mutuality
   and Possibility ... 111
   The Legacy of Children ... 111
   Observers and Observed: Embodied, Enchanted,
      and Compassionate ... 113
   BambinO: A Case Study of an Opera Composed and Performed
      for Infants ... 117

7. The Musical Legacies of Childhood and Children ... 129
   Becoming Music ... 130
   Being Present ... 130
   Alone and with Others: The Social Contexts of Musical Experience ... 132
   Making the Path: Interactions of Stability and Change over Time ... 137
   Interruption, Trauma, and the Rerouting of Musical Lives ... 144
   Empathy, Trust, and Wonder: A Pedagogy of/for Children ... 148

Epilogue: Childhoods in Flux: Considering Consequences of
a Global Pandemic ... 155
   Music as a Social Tool ... 155
   Parents as Teachers: Finding Time and Spaces for Learning ... 156
   Renewing Enchantment and Synchronicity ... 157
References ... 159
Index ... 167

Foreword

The Resonant Legacies of Childhoods and Children

In a recent video interview (https://www.youtube.com/@pennstate) where I was asked to discuss a personal passion, I talked about the joy I find in playing music. In the piece, the video producers elicited from me the kind of musical autobiography that forms the source material for much of the scholarship shared in this book. I offered that I have been a fan of popular music as long as I could remember, following the example set by my father. Born in Queens, New York, in 1922, he, along with his neighborhood friends, was drawn to the sound and spectacle of swing music. Guided by his more knowledgeable peers, he learned to play drums, found his way into a neighborhood big band, and at twenty years old was on his way to becoming a union musician. World War II then intervened. By the time I was born in the early 1960s, my father had become a veteran of the US Navy, gone through college on the GI bill, established a career as a social worker, and, so far as I know, never again was a member of a band. However, throughout my entire childhood, the southeast corner of our basement was fully occupied by his champagne sparkle Gretsch drum kit. Every weekend, without fail, he would find the time to cue up a thick stack of big band LPs on his enormous console stereo (Basie, Dorsey, Ellington, Miller, etc.) and play along for ninety minutes like the Krupa-inspired rhythm king that he had been and still was.

His influence on me was undeniable. Although I didn't begin playing music until I was in my early twenties, I did so, just like him, guided by more knowledgeable peers who urged me to give it a try. Being well aware that, famously, Paul Simonon (from the Clash) couldn't play a note when Joe Strummer thrust that telecaster bass into his hands, I was coaxed into picking up the bass guitar. Neither my dedication nor talent has proven Simononian and my first band didn't last all that long, but intermittently, throughout my life, I have found my way into rock bands. There have been long dry spells in between stints, but the formative musical experiences of my childhood and emerging adulthood have pulled me back into bands repeatedly.

When I reflect on what I love about playing in a band, I always think of my father. I am saddened by the fact that he never was able to recapture the band experience of his youth later in his life. Of course, swing music just didn't have comparable pop culture endurance of rock 'n' roll. On top of that, the logistical challenges of filling out a bandstand with the dozen or so players needed for a big band dwarfs the work it takes to stand up your standard four-piece rock outfit. Despite whatever combination of obstacles kept him from rejoining a band, I know that his individual connection to his music and his musicianship was deeply meaningful to him throughout his life. We made sure that the swing music was playing during his memorial, and I can tell you that the choicest selections from his record collection are with me still.

As you will learn from reading this book, Dr. Custodero draws a range of informative conclusions about the import of early life musical experience from her study of the retrospective musical autobiographies provided to her by the graduate music education students she has worked with over her career. She offers cogent observations on the primacy of musical activity in all our lives, reflects on how memories, especially musical memories, are made, and effectively employs the "kaleidoscope" as a metaphor for both the interdisciplinary methodologic approach she presents, and the inherent complexity of ways that individuals build their own musical identity. Though I am not a music educator, I *am* an educator, and even relative to my own field of expertise, the act of considering my (and my father's) formative years' musical autobiography has offered useful analogies and emotional resonance. As a listener and still episodic performer of music, the exercise catalyzed by my video project and sustained by writing this foreword has given me with a deeper understanding of the meaning that I find in music. The tools and perspective Dr. Custodero offers aspiring music educators will, I suspect, better prepare them to understand the complex and deeply personal context already forming in their students when they first encounter them.

Craig J. Newschaffer, PhD
Raymond E. and Erin Stuart Schultz Dean
College of Health and Human Development
Pennsylvania State University

1
Musical Beings

Childhood, Children, and Music

Musical Legacy

Music has evolved as a sonic amplification of our physical, social, and emotional human experience. We carry this legacy ontogenetically: memories of profound experiences of music in our own childhoods, and as adults in our observations of and interactions *with* children, shape us as performers, parents, and teachers. Reflection on our musical experience is crucial to our understanding of the fundamental nature of music in our lives and our approach to guiding others in musical endeavors.

Across generations and even centuries, connecting with other humans is at the core of our understanding of self and our relationship to the world. This sympathetic knowledge derives from our childhood ways of being, and it might even be said that our development as artistic adults is a "growing into" the promise of our childhoods. Such promise is realized as we attend to both the childlike characteristics within, and the children around, each of us. It is through these joint processes of introspection and interaction that we retain the ability to embody sound in movement, to embrace the unknown, to imagine the yet to be, and to engage with the content and company of everyday life with curiosity.

Indeed, children's attunement to the world reflects openness to possibility and welcomes imaginative interpretation—we are charmed by a young child's spontaneous echo of the subway bell as the doors close but wouldn't consider engaging in the behavior ourselves. As adults, we often become closed to such direct and embodied expression, having experienced the limitations of perceived social appropriateness, and developed habits of routine response. Creative professionals often look to childhood ways of being in order to recapture the vitality and fresh perspective characteristic of their youthful selves. Composer Mikis Theodorakis (2007) spoke eloquently of his childhood curiosity as "musical *genesis*" (p. 2), providing the foundation for inquiry from which his adult musicality would flourish. What are the legacies of childhood that create opportunities for us to shed the acquired baggage of adulthood and *our* musical lives? What can we learn from children about how to nurture *their* musical lives?

A contemporary and friend of Theodorakis, Manos Hadjidakis, valued the playful childlike explorations that informed his own creative process and has been quoted as saying that "wherever children are found, we are found as well" (in Miralis, 2004, p. 50), this image of shared space implying common experiences of children and composers.

Seeking commonalities and sharing meaningful interactions result in what Dissanayake (2000) refers to as mutuality: we look at children and see recognizable selves, and they do the same with us, explicitly imitating our actions in efforts to belong with us. So it is not only by reaching within and drawing upon our own early experiences that evokes musicality; it is also being with children in our roles as parents, teachers, and playmates that shares that attunement to the creative life.

The Meaning of Musical Experience

Music education research is often concerned with skill development—how children and adults learn to sing or move or play an instrument, maybe even to compose, universal truths to be applied in any context with any student, supporting educational practices inclined toward "fixing" the child. As an alternative, ethnographic researchers like Patricia Sheehan Campbell (2010), Kathryn Marsh (2008), and Claudia Gluschankof (2002) brought to the fore the voices and expressive movements of children in everyday life, demonstrating *how music means* to them.[1]

However, the application of these revelations to pedagogy has not been easily envisioned in the music education profession. Little attention is given to the music children make before we step in to instruct them, and very few teacher preparation programs address how music functions for children. Like adults, children may use music to comfort themselves, regulate their

---

[1] Here I am borrowing from John Ciardi, whose book *How Does a Poem Mean?* provides analytic tools for interpreting and understanding poetry that are applicable to other artistic media. He writes "the language of experience is not the language of classification.... The concern is not to arrive at a definition and to close the book, but to arrive at an experience" (p. 666). Asking "how" music means suggests an ongoing experiential frame of inquiry, open to spontaneity and surprise rather than a predetermined fixed list of expected responses.

body movements, or communicate with others. Except in cases of imitative dramatic play, children's music making is generally not meant to be a "skilled performance" repeated at the insistence of others outside of the realm of normal daily activity. For children, music is a way of being.

The multiple meanings and functions of music in human life suggest a variety of entry points to musical experiences. Regardless of age, skill level, or socioeconomic status, we sing, hum, chant, dance, listen, play instruments, alone and together, responding to rhythmic patterns and cues and to melodic and harmonic conventions. Whether sitting on a rocking chair or on an exercise bike, we use music to motivate action and to regulate our movement. We also are moved metaphorically by music, transported through our ability to imagine in sound. We connect to music from distant times and places stored as memories when neural circuitry is activated through auditory stimuli and familiar emotional states (Damasio, 2010). We engage with music in cathedrals, sports stadiums, and dorm rooms, in the family car, in concert halls, and in school classrooms, deepening both our knowledge of self and our sense of belonging. Making music together creates community—connections with our physical selves in time and space, converge with our abilities to feel, engaging in receptivity and expression of emotion (Turino, 2008). We seek and find meaning through shared musical identities, where preferences create affiliation, and through shared performance experiences, where we find a goodness of fit between our contributions and those of others.

Music influences our lives both explicitly and implicitly. Our hearts race or ache depending on the musical soundtracks in film, and we are constantly exposed to the ever-present pitch of modern technology, such as the hum of electrical current, yet we are not consciously aware. R. Murray Shafer (1994) has catalogued such sounds in literature throughout history and made connections with the music being composed at that time and the ambient musical environment. One of his clearest examples is the relationship between the carriage horses' hooves trotting over cobblestones, and the four-note arpeggiated accompaniment figure known as the "Alberti Bass," heard in much late eighteenth-century European music. The "clip clop" of the horseshoes is mimicked in the music:

♫ ♫ ♫ ♫.

We are also more directly influenced by music, as we consciously advantage its use for regulating physical entrainment and emotional expression or comfort (deNora, 2000). Whether compiling a playlist to accompany a run in the park or singing a lullaby with an unhappy child, we individually monitor our own and others' actions through music's organizing temporal structure and emotional evocation. Such monitoring is powerful; it has been the repertoire of revolutions and crises management. Throughout history, music has been used to unify, motivate, and guide action and emotion: nineteenth-century military drum and bugle corps led soldiers to battle, protest music echoed through the country during the civil rights demonstrations in the 1960s, and the US Congress publicly responded to the events of September 11, 2001, by standing on the Capitol steps and singing "God Bless America."

Musical experiences are ubiquitous, and as such, may go unnoticed and unexamined. Yet, music functions as both a signifier of emotional intensity, taking one more deeply *into* the moment, and as a vehicle for transcending the present, taking us out of the moment into the past, as in reminiscences of personal associations or images, or even into an anticipated future. Given the broad expanse of music in everyday life, it is important to consider its role in shaping us and the groups to which we belong (Dissanayake, 2000). In the following section, I illuminate how and why we are musical beings, how the temporal, dynamic, social, and physical properties of music are aligned with qualities of human existence, and how they are manifested in children's capabilities for embodiment.

Living in Music: Experiences of Time and Movement

Musical Time

The temporal nature of music asks us to attend over time—to be present in the moment while holding in our memory what just happened and hypothesizing what comes next. Think of hearing the performance of a piece for the first time. We connect what we are hearing based on what we know about music that sounds similar—recognition of genre-based conventions like a blues progression or sonata allegro form leads to specific expectations. Our experience is a resource for understanding the present encounter, the combination of association and immediacy serves to make an informed prediction of what comes next. Such challenge is uniquely compelling, perhaps because it mimics our lived experience of a present informed by the past and directed by our vision of the future: music requires of us a type of mindfulness that joins who we were and who we can be with what we are now.

This sense of expansion, what Stern (2004) refers to as "the present moment" (p. 3), brings a richness and fullness of experience that is unmatched in other human activity. It is the temporality of musical experience that provides impetus for being in the "now"; it requires our multisensory engagement, tapping into the physical, emotional, social, and aesthetic capacities to attend. These diverse entry points enable an immersion in the sound, a merging of action and awareness (Csikszentmihalyi, 1990), a suspension of the everyday to encounter the extraordinary (Dissanayake, 2000).

This quality of focus on the immediate context has been investigated by scholars like Levine (1998), who refers to this attention to the present as event time. He compares this to clock time in which we live by our externally generated schedules and attend to the notion of time passing, rather than being engaged with the task or with the aesthetically compelling moment. Consider the New York City subway during the evening rush. People are scurrying from one train to another, others waiting and watching the brightly lit announcement board counting down the minutes to arrival. Suddenly, the sounds of a panpipe and guitar come into consciousness, and for a moment, the clock-based perception of time becomes event-based. Although fleeting, this brief encounter with meaningful musical activity impacts, some might say enhances, the quality of lived experience.

Chances are that if you didn't notice the musicians, a child would have shown you the way—children are seeking engagement with the world most of the time. They live in event time rather than clock time, and the nature of their interpretations and engagement with musical stimuli provides dynamic and embodied representations of the event.[2]

Musical Movement

Time is one way we structure living. We speak of our relationship to time in terms of movement—it passes slowly or quickly, it is represented visually in a continuously moving radius from right to left, or digitally through change we interpret as movement. We also describe life's organizing forms and

---

[2] See, e.g., Sara Zur's (2007) study on children's musical play and clock time vs. event time in Darwin, Australia, Singapore, and New York City.

structures through observed and experienced changes suggesting movement. There is movement in our interpretation of the natural world: the sun "goes down" to turn day into night, and seasons come and go. Developmentally, we "go through" various stages (puberty, mid-life crises) and "move into" old age. Our psychological states include moods that "swing" and emotions that "run wild."

Music mimics this human predilection toward movement; taking a view of music as an analogue of the body, it becomes animated, shaped by the variety of characteristics that define it. The examples above reflect a variety of life rhythms. Musically speaking, we start with our life source, the pulsing heartbeat, as the primary organizer of rhythm, and our bipedal subdivision as foundation of meter and periodicity. Our sense of moving in space is manifested in pitch-related perceptions of melody and harmony. Melody is defined by the range and contour of its vertical ascent and descent as it moves (horizontally) through time; its linear quality suggests the individual's experience in making their life path. Harmony refers to both a single simultaneity of tones (referred to as chords or clusters in the parlance of Western music), and as a progression—a temporal sequence of these individual constructions. It provides the context for the individual's melodic path.

In addition to these mirrors of our physical experience in the world, we can consider movement as the result of interactions between these characteristics of sound. Ciardi (1959) used the concept of movement to theorize *how* a poem "means." He analyzed qualities of motion such as acceleration and resistance in the sounds of a poem, and considered how numerous elements of form including rhyme, imagery, and diction, interacted to counter the motion established by the metric regularity (or irregularity).

Western tonal music is pushed forward by dominant harmony; motion is inhibited by its resolution to tonic. Acceleration of rhythmic intensity moves us forward in time, while use of longer durations resists this force. Periodic phrasing sets up a pattern that leads to anticipation of continuity as well as variation—often the pattern is extended, creating surprise and altering our experience of movement in the piece. From Haydn's startling fortissimo chord, which halts the quiet tiptoes of pizzicato strings in his 94th "Surprise" Symphony, to Philip Glass's subtle harmonic changes that glimmer with a perpetual resonance, we experience multiple qualities of movement as we listen to music.

Except for those whimsical moments when our attunement to social mores and protocol takes leave, adults tend to internalize the movement experienced in music. Yet we can be completely enchanted by the child's freedom to respond overtly to qualities of musical movement—we look at one another and smile when a toddler begins bouncing to a beat, and share YouTube videos of children dancing, absorbed in the moment, living in the music. This seeing oneself—or one's experience—in the form of another's living body produces a synthesis of sound and sight that heightens meaning.

A 2005 interview with a former student who, at the time, was teaching jazz classes for children ages two to five, revealed his attention to this phenomenon of musical embodiment regarding his young students. In talking about his work, he offered[3]:

I learned [by] observing children . . . when they're interpreting or listening to something, it becomes like real. . . . Their whole body changes into this emotional thing. . . . I see these children listening to sounds—either my guitar or a recording—and they really become the sound. If the sound is like Charlie Parker playing fast on the sax, they are a fast saxophone. . . . There's no limit to what they can or cannot be. And they can be sound itself. . . . They make it their own . . . they take it, they listen to it and say "This is mine, I am it." (Jason, 2005)

Such embodiment is how children experience music—and how Ciardi explains the "reason a poem means." Quoting Yates, he highlights the immersive qualities of artistic engagement:

O body swayed to music, O quickening glance,
   How shall I tell the dancer from the dance?" (Ciardi [1959], p. 4)

This merging of actor and act, prompted by aural cues, is a result of the capacity of music to move us. Such music-invoked movement is a human response to the analogous relationship between sound and body; it is an artifact of culture and experience. Because we cannot always control our sonic environment, and because we cannot "listen away" in the same way we can "look away," we are susceptible to the features of what we hear. We become vulnerable to musical cues such as a driving pulse—we move in response to its power and are drawn into the rhythmic energy of entrainment, a synchrony

---

[3] Throughout this book, extended quotations by study participants will be shown in italics.

of external sound and physical movement. This is why music is often used to accompany exercise: the compelling beat of a pop tune serves as a tool for self-regulation of movement (deNora, 2000).

Movement to music is often used to help children regulate: many cultures have traditions involving parents swaying or rocking infants in their arms, laying infants across their laps and gently bouncing them on their knees, or carrying infants on their backs and walking, in each instance accompanied by singing. The singing/moving provides the regularity that can calm and comfort, improving critical systemic functions including heart rate and breathing (Trehub, 2009).

Young children use movement and music in similar ways. In a study of spontaneous music making in Taipei, Taiwan, a group of student researchers and I observed children in public places (e.g., museums, restaurants, and parks). We noted that music-related movement was recorded in 75 percent of the documented musical episodes (Custodero et al., 2006). In a later study, data were collected in New York City subways, where movement is not always welcomed; still, we found that 48 percent of the episodes involved moving (Custodero, Calì, & Donoso, 2016). Movement accompanied other musical behaviors like singing, chanting, and playing objects as instruments, both as a response to music heard and as a companion to singing.

To review, I am suggesting that we are musical beings by virtue of our movement through time. Music re-presents our physical selves, and the vocabulary we use to describe music presents intriguing evidence of our embodied experience. Our responses to music reflect these connections more explicitly, as we are moved by music both literally, as the motor cortex is activated during listening (e.g., Zatorre, Chen, & Penhune, 2007), and metaphorically, as our memories and emotions are also activated.

These experiences of time and movement create opportunities for musical interactions that contribute to human functioning through their connection to emotions. Thinking of an existential triangle of self-other-environment, music provides a means in which we can express ourselves, commune and communicate with others, and create sonic environments of safety and comfort, as well as fear and rage. Children teach us much about music and emotion, as they are particularly vulnerable to the "feeling" of music because their embodied experience of sound makes it difficult to objectify. The openness of childhood provides a lesson reflecting artistic activity: "I am it"—the merging of the dancer and the dance.

Feeling of Music: Expression, Communication, and Comfort

Music as Expression

People have used music to intensify emotional experience and to express universally personal and infinitely diverse spiritual rituals and political motives. Music has dramatic effect, playing upon our sensations of time and movement, conveying the emotional backdrop of stories in operas and movies in a stealth-like manner, remaining unknown in our consciousness yet directly playing upon our feelings.

For young children, this experience is especially intense, as I discovered early in my career. I was delivering music experiences at a Head Start preschool in Los Angeles. It was December, and I thought it would be fun to play with some pieces from The Nutcracker Suite by Tchaikovsky. I unwittingly chose "The Dance of the Sugarplum Fairy," which is in a minor key and starts with plucked strings bouncing from lower to higher registrars introducing the "tiptoeing" melody in the celeste. I imagined we could be walking carefully through the forest, moving around the classroom teachers who were to be trees, with arms posed as branches, but hadn't realized that the minor mode and timbres might call forth ominous images. We barely made it through eight bars before the class became terrified—some in tears, some cowering, others clinging to their teachers. The emotional content of the music expressed something very tangible to them; fantasy and reality were fused, and the effect was very powerful. We quickly ended the activity with a quick diversion in the drama—minus the soundtrack: "And then we all ran out of the forest and had a delicious picnic at the playground!"

Links between musical expression and emotions have historical precedence. Ancient Greece differentiated between the Apollonian harp, which represented the controlled, logical persona, and the Dionysian aulos, which represented the abandonment of reason and a celebration of the bacchanal. Likewise, the seventeenth-century Baroque doctrine of affections featured various key areas matched with specific affective states; composers could express a variety of emotions by the systematic application of the appropriate mode, and this expression could be easily identified by the audiences of the time.

Today's audiences are global, and such generalizations of feeling music are both (a) called into question through acknowledgment of musical expression as culturally defined and sanctioned, and (b) perpetuated by a movement toward a single global culture, becoming more actualized through the mass export of American/British popular music (Gebesmair & Smudits, 2001). Dual trends are evident in children's musical lives as well. There are seemingly universal practices of parental musical expression, such as the lullaby, which is sung or hummed by the adult to the child. Yet, when we studied US parents who sang to their children, we found differences in what types of songs were sung, dependent upon the adult's musical experience—for example, those who had sung in a choir were more likely to sing lullabies to their young children. In other words, they expressed themselves by accessing the conventional repertoire for infants. Alternately, those who identified as instrumentalists and those who had taken lessons were more likely to play recorded music to interact with their babies (Custodero & Johnson-Green, 2003).

Musical expression is a result of what Damasio (1999) calls "the incontrovertible correlation between the private and the public" (p. 13) in his discussion of the emotion-feeling interface. It is both based in perception, as when we receive and interpret musical expression individually, and based in behavior, as when we express ourselves musically. For young, preverbal children, musical perception and behavior are easily observed, since their expressive skills involve physical interactions—both facial expression and bodily movement—with the stimulus, and responsive vocalizations mimicking speech. These modes of expression are unfiltered and unmasked, bound by the child's developing physical and linguistic skill. Examples of children's musical response and music making charm us, evidenced by the number of internet images of children making and responding to music that have gone viral. Whether we see images of the "toddler bounce," when children stand, bending at the knees, and bob up and down to rhythmic music; or infants tearing up as their mother sings a beautiful ballad to them; or fathers playing drumming duets with their preschool child, these renderings of feelings connect us all to the significance and familiarity of shared musical experiences.

One function of music, then, is to provide a means of capturing the essence of emotion and expressing the resultant feelings. It provides a means through which we understand the expressive intention of others, and a way to vicariously share in the experience. Another related function of music is to communicate, to express specific messages that are conveyed and understood within a common culture, what Blacking (1995) referred to as a "sound group."

Music as Communication

Whereas expression is about putting forth the personal into the public, communication is a purposeful connection made with another. The sound group provides a context for musical interaction and may be considered a cultural unit that shares a musical language. Although music is sometimes considered a "universal language," the closest we may come to that superlative is in early childhood. Imagine you are holding an infant in your arms. How would you speak to her? What would your affect be? What responses would you expect? If you are like most of us, your voice would be more melodic than everyday speech, with a greater range and dramatic contour, your affect, exaggeratedly positive. You are most likely rewarded with body movement, focused eye contact, vocalizations, and a smile. This results in more of the same—a back-and-forth conversation where leader and follower roles disappear.

Such communicative experiences are at the essence of our humanity (Trevarthen & Malloch, 2016). They are overtly present in the daily lives of children from birth through adolescence and continuing, often more hidden, through adulthood and old age. In infancy, our sound group comprises our parents/caregivers and siblings with whom we offer and receive socially understood signals through expressive vocalizations, many of which seem universal across cultures (Papousek, 1996). Between the ages of three and five we begin to accrue multiple sound groups, each with an identifiable shared repertoire and set of musical practices. We have music at home, which may include siblings; family music outside the home, such as a place of worship; music at school or daycare, typically teacher-led; and music on the playground, most of which involves communicating with peers. Each of these sound groups provides resources with which children construct musical worlds. Later, in adolescence, peer groups become sound groups, and the musical language is even more specific.

These communicative groups tend to be bracketed, that is, they are discrete—see, for example, the Goth music subcultures cited on Wikipedia including gothic rock, industrial, deathrock, post-punk, darkwave, ethereal wave, and neoclassical, each with its own musical language. As in linguistic communication, the styles may be inaccessible to those without fluency. We can often make an inference about what is being communicated based on a limited knowledge of the musical language and our past experiences. We also read and interpret physical cues like facial expressions and body gestures; however, assumptions that are derived from one sound group are not necessarily transferable to another. In the classroom, the teacher-led musical communication is generally accepted by the sound group of children, although my research in preschool music settings (e.g., Custodero, 2005) suggests that the teacher may initiate activity; but it is peers who sustain it. On the playground, music making is child-initiated and maintained. It has its own fluency, and may borrow repertoire from the classroom, transforming it to suit the language of musical play—changing the words, the structure, repeating small rhythmic or melodic motifs that communicate the imaginative worlds they are building.

The influence of the setting has much to do with how sound groups are formed and who is included. When children, who are believed to be dependent upon others for repertoire, can claim that repertoire for themselves, it then can be resourced as needed—whether for expression, communication, or for comfort. The awareness of musicianship as a facilitator of agency has strong implications for how and what we teach.

Music as Comfort

As noted previously, we have used music to comfort ourselves both on the national and international stage when tragedy has occurred, as well as in intimate settings of parent-child interactions. We can create, regulate, and intensify or soothe emotional states by listening to and performing music for ourselves and with others. Children teach us how best to comfort them through responding to our efforts. As they do this, they are helping shape a repertoire of effective strategies that they can then eventually enact for themselves.

We are comforted by music for many reasons, including its organizational structures and patterns. The regularity of a steady pulse can help us gain control over our bodies, and physiologically overcome the chaos and anxiety caused by psychological and physical distress. Instead of being frustrated and sad when it's time to put the toys away, children are happy to help when the news is delivered with the "Cleanup Song." That is because the metric division of 6/8 time falls into two groups of three, a sort of "waltz inside of a march," a compelling rhythm that swings us into a comforting motion.

Another example of comforting form is in the call-and-response vocalized interactions between infants and adults. Familiarity with turn-taking structure can be a source of comfort based in realized expectations. This is borne out in research on infant-mother communication where dyadic interactions have been shown to be so synchronous that one could draw bar lines (showing metric patterns) to the shared sounds (Malloch & Trevarthen, 2009). Studies of postpartum depression have found this synchrony to be tied to wellbeing: when the mother is depressed, infant-mother interaction is not synchronous, but the synchrony returns when the diagnosis is lifted (Field, 2010). Comparable to a jazz band trading phrases, the reciprocity of being heard and responded to reflects the inter-subjectivity of sound groups.

Comfort is created not only by the shared musical language, but also by the concomitant interpersonal associations we develop with specific people as well as musical pieces that become our "go to" repertoire. The power of association with certain music is known to most of us—we can be transported to a specific setting or imagine a certain person by hearing a tune, rhythm, or chord progression. This can be comforting, especially when we initiate the sensory experience; it can be disarming when we are taken by surprise. I remember stories from my teenage piano students, who would talk of playing Beethoven's "Pathétique Sonata," feeling comforted by the expressive outlet for their inner angst. Yet, if we are feeling vulnerable, hearing that same piece can cause great discomfort, a response exemplified in the preschool children listening to Tchaikovsky.

There are many examples of children's use of music to comfort themselves. Sole's (2016) research on toddlers' pre-slumber vocalizations suggests that they often revisit familiar songs experienced that day to lull themselves to sleep or will use familiar melodies with invented words to make sense of something that may be troubling for them.

In our study of singing in families (Custodero, 2006, 2008), the mother of a three-year-old reported:

> *Then after everyone was in bed, Kylie sang "Twinkle, Twinkle Little Star" to herself, several times, too loudly for my taste. So I fussed at her that she had to stop making so much noise. And she started singing the song with sort of a humming noise and doing, I don't know what you call it, this funny thing with your lips when you go (lip trill) like that? So she did that, until she fell asleep.*

Every night, Kylie and her two siblings were individually sung to by one or both of their parents. Here, Kylie could comfort herself, using the music to evoke a feeling of being cared for, drawing upon the associations of parent-child routine, as she transitions between wakefulness and sleep. This use of music to bring the internal need to external manifestation suggests that it serves as what Winnecott (1971) referred to as a transitional object, a resource utilized by young children to bring the comfort of parent/home/safety to a less familiar environment.

The topic of music as transitional object came to the foreground in a study we did on children's music making on New York City subways (Custodero et al., 2016). Music making served as a resource which made the unfamiliar space more inhabitable: children sang familiar songs softly to themselves, made up songs based on advertisements on the subway wall, and moved and tapped to songs in their heads. These were strategies to bring familiar musical practices to the stranger-filled public space, revisiting them as aids in the transition between home and not home, the known and the unknown.

And so, we return to the public-private duality of musical experience. A final example from Kylie's mother's audio diary shows the complexities of music making in intimate, communal settings:

> *Kylie brought the little . . . electronic toy piano thing out into the foyer of our house. She said, "OK, now I'm going to sing my last song to you." She sang this lo-o-o-ng thing, where she was playing piano, you know, just punching the random keys, and she was singing, . . . And it was the long expressive thing, where she was talking about her whole day. She talked about how she missed her mom during the day, and then she was happy when her mom came home. She talked about how she was sad because she wanted her beautiful day, and the rain kept coming and it wouldn't go away, and she couldn't have her beautiful day because of the rain, and all this stuff. Very lengthy, expressive, thing she was doing, she was singing, while she played the piano. And of course, I was thinking, well, you know, Kylie's a genius. OK, that's it (Laughter).*

In this example, the improvisatory, narrative nature of the song seems to indicate a clear expressive function for Kylie, who was purposeful about communicating with her mother. Her intentional expression brings comfort to both singer and listener, resulting in an intimate sharing enjoyed by each participant.

Before We Teach

In this chapter, I established a foundation for considering music education in direct correspondence to the human experience of time, movement, and intention. There is much evidence for the primacy of musical activity in our lives, and although often ubiquitous, it positions music learning as relative to our social, physical, and sonic environments. Additionally, the awareness of music's function in the expression of emotion, in communicative engagement, and in the delivery of comfort and self-care provides insight into what and how music means. In acknowledging these roles of music as a catalyst for individual agency and a tool for human flourishing, we must strive to enact pedagogical practices that reflect such musical positioning and function.

I propose that attending to childhood experiences in music is key to our understanding of what and how we teach all students. Musical encounters in our own childhoods establish cultural values and practices (e.g., Trehub, 2009), which interact with ever-changing affordances across the lifespan. In the next chapter, I discuss the interdisciplinary lenses used to address the patterns and variability of lived childhoods. Using models from Psychology, Music Education, and Cultural Anthropology, I prepare the reader for subsequent analyses of musical autobiographies culled from over 200 music education graduate students. In this second of two introductory chapters, I examine the characteristics of memory and consider how reflection brings musical legacies to consciousness.

This overview is followed by three chapters that explore questions about how music means within broadly conceived developmental contexts: (1) early childhood musical experiences, which usually involve relationships with family and/or extensions of the family into neighborhoods, and set in place dispositions for music making; (2) the evolution of identities in music as listener, performer, and instrument player/singer, while striving to match dispositions with opportunities—most commonly occurring in middle childhood and early adolescence; and (3) the disruption of trajectories and subsequent resilience and/or renewal of musical lives. These stories are not necessarily linear. They are meant to generate the reader's own recollections and provoke a process of self-reflection on how the musical legacies of our own childhoods live in us now and contribute to our present selves and to our possible future, both as musicians and as music educators.

Observing children as they play freely with and through music reminds us of how music means not only for them, but for us as well. In the penultimate chapter I address how interacting with children expands our capacities to live musically and to cultivate a musical life. Our foundational, embodied knowledge of music is readily experienced in our childhoods, and it is being in the presence of children that keeps us mindful of this aesthetic promise.

We are musical beings, and by tracing our own dynamic musical histories, we gain awareness about the coherence of our present circumstances including our own interpretations and practices around subjective issues such as challenge, change, agency, and beauty. Musical encounters *with children* allow us to see the delight in discovery of what to us has become mundane. By making the familiar strange, by viewing the everyday as special (Dissanayake, 1995), we can renew a sense of wonder and curiosity that fuels creative and ethical work. Before we teach, these legacies of children and childhood have much to tell us.

2

"Prelude to a Method"

Memories, Music, and Childhood

Introduction

This chapter title pays homage to Edith Cobb, whose 1977 posthumously published book, *The Ecology of Imagination in Childhood*, begins with these four words: "Prelude to a Method." In her thoughtful articulation of adult artistry, she uses autobiographical musings of major literary and philosophical figures "to explore further the role of childhood in personal history and to examine afresh the development of the little human animal learning to transcend his [sic] biological nature in order to acquire a cultural heritage" (p. 18). Cobb was a friend of Margaret Mead, who wrote an introduction to the book where she traces the author's interdisciplinary evolution of thought and describes her method as a "mosaic" made of "quotations, observations of children, responses to projective techniques, and autobiographical material" (p. 9).

With this book, I am using an analogous strategy, one that employs similar materials and processes to *examine afresh* the significance of childhood's role in the development of a musical heritage. To follow Mead's interpretation of method as mosaic, however, is to assume a fixed position for each of these contributing modes of evidence. I prefer the image of a kaleidoscope, in which the colors and shapes shift positions, revealing possibilities of meaning and connections that may surprise.

Reading Cobb is an essential part of my own scholarly autobiography; her message regarding the links between creative adults and the inherent imagination and curiosity of children resonated deeply with my experiences as performer, composer, teacher, and researcher. I was traveling across the country to a conference when I encountered her writing for the first time and remember quite clearly the sense of elation I felt: it was reminiscent of the mutuality (Dissanayake, 2000) described in the first chapter, where one senses a recognizable self, in my case, in the writing of another. She finds the essence of human experience to be revealed in the child's interactions with the world, citing their proclivities toward sensory perception and a drive fueled by an attitude of wonder and fearlessness. She writes, "Childhood's willing acceptance and enjoyment of the muck and mire of life completes this power of creating mutual relations with the total environment and further empowers understanding of all levels of controlled thought in later life" (Cobb, p. 31).

Subsequently, I have followed Cobb's lead, learning much by attending to children's use of music in everyday life and to the autobiographical reflections on musicians' childhoods. In my work as a professor, I have adopted the practice of asking music education graduate students to write their own music autobiographies, to tell their stories, as one way to connect their teaching with their own development and learning. This process provides insights into how and why we may respond to perceived challenges in our current teaching environments. For example, many recollections reveal our previously unexamined replications of past models we have experienced—we often "teach as we were taught." In this way, narrating our musical histories becomes a method of inquiry into who, why, and what we teach, guided by questions such as: How are children musical? What is a musical childhood? What are the legacies of our own childhoods? How might they affect our teaching, creating, and researching?

In this chapter I present the methods and resources used to address these issues. Building on the embodied experiences and social-emotional functions of music described in Chapter 1, I make a case for the significance of recalling our past experiences of childhood and our awareness of childhood ways of knowing as means to understanding our musical and pedagogical selves.

Childhood and the Historical Self

Characteristics of Autobiographical Reflection

We each have an autobiographical story to tell, one that is constructed through the emotional contexts in which we've experienced life events, both momentous and routine. The process of reflection seems to awaken a curiosity in the historical self: our stories tell of perceived pathways and

"PRELUDE TO A METHOD" 19

roadblocks that temporarily define our fleeting present, simultaneously projecting this historical self into an imagined future.

Who we are and our vision of who we will be are dependent upon our interpretation of what we were—the ways in which we recollect our past experiences. We make meaning of why and how we think, act, produce, and socialize now through understanding what has shaped us before. These understandings are not ready-made or even stable, but constructed and ever-changing, based on the layers of interactions between self and context. Each time we recollect, our interpretation of that memory may change based on a specific setting, where people and place and the compelling call to elaborate or "make special" (Dissanayake, 2013) all have consequences for how and what we remember.

The excerpt below from a music student's autobiography suggests that music was a socializing experience for her, one from which she derived great joy:

> *I remember my mother washing my hair and my sister's hair in the bathtub and singing "I'm going to wash that man right out of my hair." My father used to sing a song, "There were three jolly coachmen, they went to the English tavern," and he would make our dolls and stuffed animals dance to the tune. Around the same time, my parents took us camping. In the car, the tapes (8 tracks!) were John Denver and Peter Allen. I remember loving this music, "Rocky Mountain High," "Sunshine on my Shoulder," "I Go to Rio." Perhaps I have especially vivid memories of this music because it evokes memories of a time when my whole family was together, singing together. (Hillary, 2004)*

I have an empathetic response to these experiences as I read them, as they bring to mind similar experiences in my own life. The author gives details, creating clear images of the parents' ubiquitous use of music, and chooses strong language ("I remember loving this music") to describe her emotional state in the experience. She goes on later in the narrative:

> *During the pre-K period, my sister and I enrolled in a modern dance class held at a nearby temple. My parents have a film of us at the dance concert*
>
> *... it seems like the teacher gave us a lot of freedom to dance as we pleased, because no one in the video is doing exactly the same thing. But, at the same time there is some semblance of structure, as we are all circling the same way at the same time. This image illustrates how individuality can be expressed*

within the context of a community, values that I plan to emphasize in the classroom. (Hillary, 2004)

Here, the author explicitly reveals that her own narrative informs her decision about what kind of teacher she wants to be. This transfer of autobiographical to the pedagogical frame speaks to the significance of doing this work with educators.

For those of us who teach, awareness of what drives our practice is crucial to our ability to enact a responsive pedagogy. We need to cultivate our reflective capacities and develop empathetic sensitivity to the contexts and content of student learning by looking within. By looking at memories of our own musical childhoods, we may be better able to critically examine why we do what we do.

Documenting Perspectives on Childhood: The Autobiographers

To examine the construct of a historical self, I report on the results of an ongoing study of over 200 musical autobiographies written by music education graduate students as the first assignment in a course on children's musical development. Students are given two weeks to write five to seven pages and organize their stories chronologically in four periods: early childhood, elementary school years, secondary education, and young adulthood. They are asked to discuss any meaningful musical relationships and are encouraged to include the impact of musical works, places, and events in both formal and informal settings. (See Table 2.1.)

Table 2.1 Music autobiography assignment

---

(1) Tell your musical life story in these stages:
  - Early childhood, from birth through preschool
  - Elementary school years
  - Secondary school years
  - High school graduation to the present
  - Tell about people, places, events that were important to you musically.
(2) Do you remember certain songs or pieces of music that were especially meaningful? What made them so?
(3) Think about your formal (in-school) as well as informal (with friends and family, by yourself) experiences.

This research on our memories of childhood is not concerned with the accuracy of the stories so much as with **how childhood memories are constructed and how those constructions define us as musical adults**, especially those of us who have interactions with children. Additionally, it is important to note that this is a purposeful sample, focused on autobiographies of experienced and fledgling educator-musicians who have chosen an urban Ivy League setting for their post-graduate education. However, the group is not demographically homogeneous—there is variation in country of origin, race,[1] age, musical experience, socioeconomic status, gender, and sexual orientation. In the examination and presentation of the data, I resisted making grand claims and include exemplars as well as outliers to honor the complex and idiosyncratic nature of the stories. When possible and relevant, I offer brief biographical information on the student authors.

Critically examining our own childhoods and the influential relationships with people, sound, and pedagogical conditions defining various times of life can produce an intrapersonal construction of why we are and who we are musically.[2] This recognition of our historical selves can serve to inform our pedagogical decisions: we can see classrooms and studios as empathetic contexts, rigged for the construction of meaning through musical experiences that are relevant, authentic, and shared.

Reconstructing and Remembering

Placing ourselves in historical context gives a temporal perspective on our development as musical beings and encourages us to find connections between who we were and who we are. Our memories are constructed stories, taking on a meaning based on the circumstances in which they are remembered. They are not necessarily always accurate, yet they serve to clarify values and to aid in a definition of self as musician and teacher.

---

[1] In 2018, based on self-identification, the institution's student body comprised 20% international students from seventy-seven different countries; of those remaining, 13% identified as African American, 13% Asian American, 14% Latinx, 52% Caucasian. Percentages are rounded up or down.

[2] Looking to childhood for precursors to engagement in disciplined professions is not a new idea. See, e.g., Anna Neumann's 2009 study on mid-career college professors from a variety of fields who often report an early fascination with their subject matter.

Memory and Emotion

Autobiographical memory is a type of long-term memory—an amalgamation of facts and events. Daniel Siegel defines it as "the way past events affect future function" (1999, p. 24). He writes about the importance of the emotional context of experience, as the brain's organizing process is emotional arousal. His catchphrase is "Neurons that fire together wire together"; in other words, the emotional conditions in which we experience an object or situation become associated with the content of that experience. The firing and wiring create patterns that become part of our repertoire of meaning making and continue to shape our responses throughout the lifespan. Emotional messages we receive in childhood become memories influencing adulthood, mitigated by recall and our abilities to reflect.

Literature on autobiographical memory suggests it serves multiple functions in our human development. Rasmussen and Berntsen (2009) refer to three types: directive, that is, remembering instrumental and guiding behaviors that protect us from negative consequences; self-conceptual, vis-à-vis our present identity and its continuity over time; and social, in terms of communication and bonding. In general, musical autobiography is mostly associated with the second and third types and can have negative or positive consequences based upon the emotional conditions in which our musical experiences occur. When we claim: "I'm a jazz lover" or "I used to play trumpet," we identify not only with experiences of music representing specific skills and knowledge; we also affirm our belonging to a group with common interest and proclivities.

> *My preschool and elementary school years were influenced mainly by my musical experiences at church and home. I'm Seventh-Day Adventist, so we went to Sabbath School and CradleRoll (for the tiny tots). CradleRoll was wonderful! It's ALL about the music! Just song after song, complete with toys and body movement. We were rarely in our little seats during the hour. I love to sing. And I loved to sing especially as a child. (Jeanine, 2004)*

This example of a "self-conceptual" memory places the writer in a group and claims an identity as a musical member of her church that began in early childhood. All too often, I hear claims of "non-musician" identities, from people who have been silenced by a music teacher in their early years. Les Paul, the inventor of the electric guitar who performed into his nineties, was told by a childhood piano teacher that he should not waste his parents' money on lessons (O'Donnell, 2013). We owe a debt of gratitude to his mother, who ignored the warning and supported his curiosity and desire to play "by ear" rather than read the notes.

When considering memories and their associations with emotions, Rasmussen and Berntsen found several characteristics that are also evident in the musical autobiographies examined. Negative memories tended to be directive (teaching what not to do) and more subjectively distant; they were also more accurate. Positive memories contained more details about the context of an event than did the negative memories and were reported twice as often. The researchers make a case for the evolutionary power of positive memories, as they support wellbeing, and counter the depression often associated with negative memories.

A team of researchers led by Alf Gabrielsson (2011) examined strong experiences with music (SEM) over several decades, with participants ranging from thirteen to ninety-one years of age. The data are a collection of over 1,000 personal stories about musical events and encounters, many evoking strong vicarious emotions in the reader. Instructions were to "Describe in your own words the strongest (most intense, most profound) experience with music you have ever had" (p. 7). Ten percent of the experiences shared were recollected from childhood, mostly between the ages of eight and twelve. Thematic groups for childhood experiences included security/safety and closeness; absorbed, moved to wonderment, struck, overwhelmed; music for the first time; listening over and over; special days; and playing alone. This long-term study demonstrates the significance of autobiographical recollection—rather than the documentation of factual events; researchers were interested in how these storied histories reflect the current meaning of individuals' musical experiences.

Memory, Truth, and Values

In his book *Pieces of Light*, Charles Ferneyhough (2012) discusses memory as a reconstructive process in which the interpreted past is more a reflection of the self than it is an accurate reflection of history. Memory is a mental construction that is created in the moment according to the demands of the present. He writes, "When you have a memory, you don't retrieve something that already exists, fully formed—you create something new" (p. 7). This may be especially true for memories of childhood. When we consider our own memories of that time, we may begin to understand their recursive power, how they change upon recollection over time, and how such stories become a part of family folklore. The early, more implicit memories, stored as sensory images and feelings are a bit of a mystery, which a student reflected upon:

> *My mother stands over me, peering into the crib and singing the lullaby "Winkin, Blinkin, and Nod," her long hair bathed in moonlight, her voice high and sweet. Yet again, these cannot be entirely accurate, as my mother's hair has always been much shorter than this memory tells me. How then, can this memory seem so distinct and clear, yet also be so wrong? (Berkley, 2012)*

Recall the research of Rasmussen and Berntsen (2009), who found that positive memories have more contextual detail yet tend to be less accurate than negative memories. Since positive memories are recalled twice as often as negative memories, perhaps they are more vulnerable to the changes that occur upon retelling, like a psychological "tall tale."

Damasio (2010) refers to memory as the curator of values. Given the relevance of such interpretive recollection to our meaning making, examining musical autobiographies can provide a way to interpret the legacy of childhood, to demonstrate how our current beliefs are represented in memories. This is true not only for those who deliver music instruction, but also for those making policy decisions affecting student curriculum and access to artistic resources. Goals 2000: The American Education Act was a federal project that included the establishment of national standards and was touted by music education advocates as a victory for the arts as core subjects. It was signed in 1994 by then president Bill Clinton. Although not causal, one could surmise that as an award-winning high school saxophone player, his memories of music making including pep band, marching band, and performing as a jazz trio member informed his dedication to the arts. It had curated his values.

Environments, Development, and Disposition

Ecologies with and of Music

Where and with whom we engage defines the nature of our experience, fusing the emotional and perceptual with action, and creating a conjoined

"PRELUDE TO A METHOD" 25

memory. Cobb's reference to the ecology of imagination suggests that the interaction between child and environment is led by the child's need to make sense of their world, undertaken with an attitude of curiosity and possibility. She speaks of "participating in otherness while retaining a sense of one's own ego-world identity" (1977, p. 22). Here is how one of the students made sense of his world, growing up in Korea:

> *My family had a house near the mountainside in a suburban town. We had a garden and animals. I had the privilege of listening to the sound of birds and insects, the sound of a brook, and the wind blowing through leaves of the trees. All of the sounds of nature mingled together, it seemed to me a perfect harmony. It fascinated me so. I used to wake up to the black rooster we raised, and I came home from the playground at dusk, hearing the sound of [the] bell ringing from the nunnery. My interest in different timbres of sound began during that time. Music played through the record player and the natural sounds of the four seasons appealed to me differently. My imagination developed with them. (Soyoung, 2004)*

This memory of childhood encompasses the natural ecology, which helped structure and characterize his world.

A few years after Cobb's publication was released, Bronfenbrenner (1979) introduced his landmark theory of ecological systems, which considers multiple concurrent sites of influence on the child's experience. He writes that it involves the scientific study of the progressive, mutual accommodation between an active, growing human being and the changing properties of the immediate settings where the developing person lives, as this process is affected by relations between these settings and the larger contexts in which the settings are embedded.

Using a systems approach to examine childhood development acknowledges the nested contexts of home, school, neighborhood, and even nation states as environments that influence behaviors and outcomes (see Figure 2.1). In considering the larger impact of state policies on children, I am reminded of one early autobiography (from around 2000) that was especially poignant, written by a student who had grown up during the cultural revolution in China. Unfortunately, I do not have a copy of the original document, but I remember being filled with emotion while reading it. She told about how all things representing Western European culture were removed from her family home, save the grand piano that was too large to

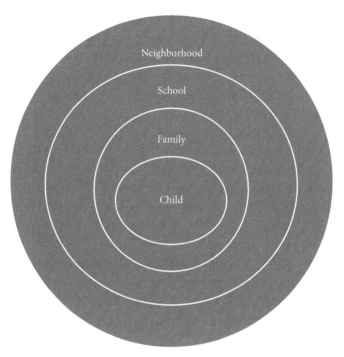

Figure 2.1 Embedded ecologies of childhood musical experience (after Bronfenbrenner, 2001; and Ilari, 2017)

fit through the doorway. Although she and her brother were admonished to never play it, she recalls stuffing towels in the small opening between the floor and the bottom of the door to stifle the quiet clandestine sounds they would make on the instrument when left alone while their parents were at work.

This was a very idiosyncratic example, but it has remained an iconic image for me representing the interactions between the power of ecological circumstance and the compelling nature of musical activity. Although the stories in this book come from people whose parents, for the most part, had the ability and interest to provide them with musical instruments and lessons, not all the participants had this advantage—there are several stories of difficulty and frustration over a lack of opportunity and access (see Chapter 5). Despite variations in economic and cultural background, there are common threads running through the narratives of people who chose a career involving music education.

Patterns of Influence

In his later rethinking of the ecological theory as *bio*ecological, Bronfenbrenner postulated that the interactions between processes (in our case, music making), person, context (e.g., family, friends, sociocultural settings), and time (historical-political and lifespan) were all crucial to human development (Tudge et al., 2009). Looking at the social and physical settings across the lifespan in autobiographies of music education graduate students, several trends became clear. The most informative reads of the data include intersections of lifespan phases and contextual themes. Memories involving early childhood had most to do with the cultural concept of family, including parents, grandparents, siblings, and extensions into wider groups of kin. Music was often a key communicative entry into relationship.

Expressions of disposition and musical identity most often surfaced in memories of middle childhood and in the context of school and peers. Claims to specific musical identities were linked narratively with epiphanies regarding performing and listening. Strong memories of disruption, renewal, and resistance occurred mainly in later adolescence and early adulthood. The last category includes both *disruptions in musician identity and trajectory*—often repaired by a change in teacher, instrument, or career that renewed and/or reinvented the musical path—and *disruptions in personal lives*, for which music served to aggravate or mend.

Although they are presented here as a developmental sequence, these patterns of influence are not meant to be bound by age-related limitations and are not completely discrete. We draw upon relationships throughout our musical lives. Dispositions are observable from birth (McAdams, 2015) and exert influence in our musical lives before middle childhood. They are closely linked to how we deal with emotions—we are taught early on how music can comfort, express, and communicate, as a tool for mediating disruption. Perhaps the most universal pattern we can trace across autobiographies is change: our identity changes over time because of our experiences and the ever-shifting contexts in which we live.

Coherence and Continuity

In addition to finding similarities running through the collection of autobiographies, there were also ontogenetic dispositions that marked coherence and continuity within individuals. My own musical autobiography is a mix of strong memories and well-spun family mythology and has identifiable threads of such consistencies. I remember someone giving our family an electric organ when I was about six, and I spent much time "finding" songs I knew on it. As a result, my grandmothers each chipped in $100 for an upright piano, and I started lessons (with a thirteen-year-old teacher). That first discovery orientation to making music has been a constant throughout my lifetime; I spent countless hours of my adolescence finding melodies to play over chord charts of popular songs and engaging in "piano karaoke," that is, playing along with recordings.

I remember music as a social phenomenon: meeting with friends and playing piano while we sang in the living room "cabarets," as well as joining band and choir at school. Playing with a rock band was my ultimate fantasy; however, because very few females were invited to join that party in the 1970s, I had to wait until my fiftieth birthday to finally play in a garage (actually, an apartment) band. My teaching and scholarship have been and continue to be guided by the notion of discovery and invigorated by being with others—by looking at my musical past, I can see more clearly who I am today and how I came to be.

This same coherence can be detected in many of the collected autobiographies. For example, we can hear an effort to cohere childhood to adulthood in this reflection on a teaching disposition emanating from an experience of a preschool dance class that appeared earlier in the chapter: "This image illustrates how individuality can be expressed within the context of a community, values that I plan to emphasize in the classroom." It should be noted that claims of coherence were not always positive—some students had difficulties making connections to their past or were unhappy with the opportunities lost.

The kaleidoscope serves as a metaphor for understanding how combinations of memories, present experiences, and projection of future opportunities may coalesce into a discernable order reflecting a sense of self and a musical identity. At its best, this sense of self is both *individually coherent* (noting similar dispositions of a person over their lifespan) and *continuously evolving over time*, responding to patterns of influence within social settings, changing developmental and sociocultural trends, and musical contexts. As we turn the kaleidoscope, we can see permutations of possibility in how musical lives are constructed, bringing a thoughtfulness to the cultivation of our own and others' musical experiences.

Kaleidoscopic Turns: Seeing through New Eyes

Adults' Encounters with Children's Music Making

Children's spontaneous musical behaviors are often interpreted as stemming from a coveted sense of freedom and an openness to prospective opportunities for action that come from "not knowing." The example below shows how composers, in this case, Elaine Barkin, value the newness and discovery that can come with naivete. She is speaking to a group of composers about an improvisational event:

> The original concern was not to find yet another way to compose music but to find a way to be an inhabitant in a world of music . . . whose content reflects the shared experiences of its participants, interacting with and supporting one another, where the search is for community rather than audience; where technique, as it is usually understood, is neither a necessity nor a virtue; where conventional musical abilities are neither required nor prohibited; where idiosyncrasies and so-called imperfections are permissible. (Barkin, 1989, p. 2)

To be awestruck by the ordinary and curious about the unknown brings about a certain reverence for subject matter that is generative. For young children, life is filled with discovery; the ability to maintain such an orientation creates a disposition for perpetuating attention and action. This drive to discover often leads to risk-taking, which is considered a crucial part of innovative art making. When children play together, the rules are temporary, convenient, and established through peer consensus. Such attention to the quality of experience shuns the idea of bounded interpretations and reflects a spirit of openness, with focus on the evolving play.

In addition to a yearning to appropriate the child's abilities to let go of self-judgment and to attend to moments of creation, we also find a certain sense of nostalgia and amazement that these small creatures can do things we do—like beating a drum or imitating a sound. There is something that evokes a sympathetic compassion and delight when we witness such engagement; for proof of this one only needs to look at social media sites to see indications of what the populace deems watchable. I did a random search on YouTube for "Babies sing and dance" and up came a twelve-minute video featuring an international collection of 10–20-second excerpts featuring the dancing moves of infants. It had been posted eight months earlier and had 7.5 million views.

We draw upon our affiliations with children's ways of being, in models of thought involving curiosity and wonder that, when retained or reinstated in adult lives, can lead to creativity, problem-solving, and innovation. We generally assume adults serve as models for children's behavior and that children are "in process" beings or "adults in waiting." What would happen if we were to turn the kaleidoscope to examine what attunement to children's use of music does for adult musicians, composers, parents, and educators? I offer two models for analysis, one concerning the mutual recognition of adult and child, which supports the idea of child as agent in relationship, and a second model based on the ways we respond to children as a source of enchantment and how that response supports our ethical propensity for doing good. I draw from my own personal interviews with composers and musicians to demonstrate how characteristics present in children are valued and intentionally borrowed.

Kaleidoscopic Design

First used in 1817, the word "kaleidoscope" is from the Greek words "kal" (meaning beautiful) and "eido" (meaning shape) + scope, meaning to view. According to the online etymology dictionary, it translates to "observer of beautiful forms." In the final section of this prelude to a method, I present three disciplinary lenses through which we can view the shared musical stories and experiences as beautiful forms. Working backward, I start with a social science perspective that includes a formalized list, configured through the coding of autobiographical interview transcripts. I compare those to my research from the music education field, and look to Edith Cobb's contributions as well, to provide a nuanced range of interpretive possibilities that will figure into subsequent analyses in the remainder of this book.

Dan McAdams's work on personality development provides a psychological view. He compiled a list of seven "Common Dimensions of Narrative Identity Coded in Life-Story Accounts" (2015, p. 265), which functions as a guide to conceptualizations that were accessible from autobiographical data. In his own research, participants are asked to outline their life stories, tell about "key scenes" in their lives, and consider the motivation, values, and dispositional traits associated with past events. Table 2.2 features these

Table 2.2 Cross-disciplinary perspectives on dimensions of autobiographical accounts

	McAdams (2015)	Cobb (1977)	Custodero
Author			
Field	Developmental Psychology	Creativity and Childhood Studies	Music Education
Data Sources	Key Scenes Life Stories	Biographies Autobiographies of Novelists, Poets, Philosophers, Scientists	Autobiographies of Music Education Students and Composers
Focus	Personality Self	Imaginative Self	Musical/Pedagogical Self
Dimensions	Agency	Plasticity of Response to Environment	Agency
	Communion	Compassionate Intelligence	Belonging
	Redemption	Wonder	Renewal
	Contamination	Permanent Norms	Disruption
	Coherence	Biocultural Continuum	Coherence
	Complexity	Creative Evolution	Kaleidoscopic Turn
	Meaning Making	World Making	Meaning Making

dimensions of self-based themes that have recurred consistently in the literature, side by side with corresponding dimensions in the subject-specific musical stories I present. Returning to the original catalyst for this work, I juxtapose the psychological and musical with Edith Cobb's multidisciplinary perspective on the genius of childhood and its value in understanding the creative process.

Looking across the rows, we can see both similarities and differences, some subtle, some more pronounced. McAdams's first dimension is Agency, referring to the extent to which we feel empowered to act on our own, and to effect change in a situation. This is important in the music stories as well. From Cobb, we find descriptions of the child's intuitive state as agentic, as in her descriptions of Plasticity of Response. Children respond when they sense an invitation to interact with attractive properties of the environment; this action is propelled by the child and is malleable depending on the physical and social attributes of the context.

Communion is described as showing and/or receiving feelings of intimacy and care, along with a sense of belonging, and is quite powerful in the musical accounts across the lifespan. Cobb spoke of the child's communion with the world as a Compassionate Intelligence, evolving from the reciprocity of the mother-child relationship, as a nurturing sense of belonging, of feeling at one with humanity. She writes:

> If cultural attitudes could be shifted toward a recognition of human desire to exercise a compassionate intelligence, not only as tool and method, but also as the chief human survival function, we would, I believe, find ourselves capitalizing on the human impulse to nurture, cultivate, and extend this vast potential. (1977, p. 111)

Redemption, when something negative has a positive outcome, and its reverse, Contamination, when a positive experience is somehow sullied or devalued, were also present in most of the life stories of music students. I refer to them as Renewals, which requires acknowledgment of a deeper past, and Disruptions, which emphasizes the change in pathways. I believe Cobb sees Wonder as redemptive in that it begins with an admission of not knowing, an uncomfortable state for many adults, and is rewarded with new knowledge (and new questions). Cobb is adamant about how the establishment of Permanent Norms contaminates the creative process, which has ramifications for the design and implementation of teaching strategies.

McAdams's Coherence dimension comprises thematic structural organization, causal relationships, and the integration of emotional responses, all of which apply to the music autobiographies as well. Because of the pedagogical questions I am asking, I am also looking at the coherence of their life histories to their teaching philosophy and practice. Cobb's concept of the Biocultural Continuum suggests there is a coherent relationship between the natural world and the cultural world. Emphasizing our "musical being-ness" she writes:

> We are compositions being performed . . . and this permits a scoring that can be recorded technically at differing levels and rhythmic rates, such as heart, pulse, or metabolic action patterns. But at the level of culture, both rhythm and form are translated and transformed into cultural systems of meaning. (1977, p. 60)

This coherence of the natural and cultural worlds is suggested in the autobiography from the student who grew up near a mountainside in suburban Korea, listening to the soundscape. Later in his story, he writes of coming to New York and hearing a wide variety of live music, including traditional Korean music: "Finding my own people's sound far from my own country excites me as much as the nature did when I was a little boy."

Complexity is a dimension of narrative that involves many (often conflicting) plots and characters and requires autobiographers to organize the seemingly disparate pieces into a collage of relationship. This is the kaleidoscopic turn, initiating change in the existing pattern to reveal multiple possibilities and new associations; in the music autobiographies these occurred as children matured, usually due to some disruption or new opportunity. Cobb alludes to complexity in her discussion about Creative Evolution, and how as adults we can reclaim the creative, embodied processes experienced in our childhoods as a way of finding new connections.

Meaning making is the goal in my pedagogical use of autobiography. The psychological perspective equates meaning making with learning something or gleaning a message resulting from an encounter. Cobb refers to world making—a more intensive interpretation that honors the agency of children in their own learning. In the musical life-stories we can see students grapple with the correspondences between their past recollections, current identity, and future paths. It is this inquiry that I follow in the next three chapters.

3

Forming Relationships

Music in Early Childhood

Accessing and Sharing Memories

What musical memories have individuals and their family members constructed over time? In these autobiographical recollections of musical experiences in the early childhood period, there were memory issues with which to contend, one of which was that such memory is explicit. Explicit memories only occur when we have developed a sense of self and have the representational tools to name the experiences, usually not until about three years of age (Siegel, 1999). To write about their very early experiences, many of the graduate students consulted an informed source, most often their parents and/or older siblings.

> *Speaking to my mother and brother over the past two weeks has allowed me to discover a great deal about my childhood I would have never recalled otherwise. I was under the impression that for the most part, my musical exposure and interest did not begin until the age of four or five, when in fact it was much earlier than that. (Jenna, 2012)*

Once memories were roused for the individual, they often offered surprises that invited new understandings and provoked additional recollection:

> *My musical memories from early childhood were buried deep inside of me until the conversation between my mother and I wakened them. I learned that my father used to play guitar and sing lullabies, folk songs, as well as his own invented melodies to me when I was still a baby. This is rather surprising because he seems to be much more quiet and serious [sic] than my mother, who loves to laugh, sing, and tell stories. When I was little, she often joined my father and the two enjoyed performing a duet for their baby girl. Although my own memories were more filled with the bedtime stories told by my mother,*

her description of the duet somehow reminded me of one particular night: I was crying fiercely and they had to hold me in their arms and walk along the quiet street (to not to disturb our neighbors next door). I could almost recall the dimmed orange color of the light on the quiet street along with my mother's tender whisper and my father's rich baritone. Although [they don't] sing duets in front me now, they often sing along with TV music. I somehow miss those family moments when we were all united by the magic of music. Ever since I came to the United States to study from the age of eighteen, the opportunities to get together with my parents became even more precious. I think to have a family singing event is a good choice once we get back together again during the summers. (Siyuan, 2015)

However, personal childhood musical recollections are sometimes irretrievable; older witnesses are either no longer living or have a definition of music that may not include the playful melodic and rhythmic interactions of family life typical in many early childhoods. This was a source of frustration for some students and produced evidence of the power of perceived personal history to influence belief systems, especially around self-image. In this next excerpt, one woman writes in a stream of consciousness style, giving us a glimpse into her self-doubt:

In class last week, we broke into small groups to discuss our salient early musical memories. The professional musicians, singers and teachers surrounding me rattled off numerous warm memories as I tried my hardest to recall just one. Anything would have been sufficient. However, nothing came to mind beyond memories of me digging for bugs under rocks or hauling around my sketchpad. I had no memorable early memories surrounding music. Perhaps that is why I never excelled in formal musical training....

I often get songs trapped in my head and silently sing them throughout the day, as I'm sure many people do. So how did I develop from a void of musical memories to a grown-up who puts music in toys for children as a living?...

Since I couldn't pull up any particularly memorable early musical experiences . . ., I enlisted my parents for help. My mother offered, "Well, you always had a sketchbook with you." I had to probe further. Finally, she revealed that she played the piano and sang to me quite a bit when I was a young child. Apparently, I would cover my ears and tell her it hurt. She'd pat the piano bench next to her and ask me to come join her. I'd shake my head and leave the room. Either I had no innate musical interest, I was overwhelmed by over stimulation, or my mother had a horrendous voice. Or maybe I did. When I asked my mother about my dearth of musical memories, she told me that I would never sing as a child, even when encouraged. She said that she thinks someone told me I had a terrible voice, because when prompted to sing I would respond by saying, "I can't sing." I don't know who may have put me on that path, but it's sad to think how much influence another person's negative opinion has on a developing child.

I have no doubt that I sang "Itsy Bitsy Spider" with my mom and bopped my body and head to beats like most toddlers and preschoolers. I just don't have any particular recollections. My father played the piano brilliantly when I was young, and both he and my aunt would play often. So, I definitely grew up surrounded by music, but apparently didn't particularly take to it at a young age. Although I attended a Montessori preschool, I don't recall any particular musical events. I remember acting out scenes from Star Wars, learning the French word for "green beans" (haricots verts), enjoying naptime on my animal-print blanket, and having a glue war with another table during arts and crafts. But no singing, no instruments, no music. Maybe I suffer from musical amnesia. (Sara, 2004)

Here, the writer is working at making sense of her perceived lack of recall, believing it is a personal deficit, rather than considering alternative hypotheses. She does remember her father's piano playing. And unlike her classmates, who were mostly performing musicians, she has probably had fewer opportunities to recall her own performative experiences, making those memories less accessible, especially those that occurred before explicit memories are stored.

The memories shared by her mother about her not singing could be due to a limited interpretation of what constitutes a song—singing is often used to accompany movement or pretend play, so is ubiquitous and perhaps not easily untangled from everyday existence. There is also the issue of how "encouragement" to sing is received by a young child. Music making can be very private and intimate for many children (van Manen & Levering, 1996), purposely used for self-comfort or regulation and not meant to be shared with adults. As I have seen in my own observational research (e.g., Custodero, Cali, & Diaz Donoso, 2016) as well as the review of many observations reported by my students, children's spontaneous singing often stops when they become aware that they are the focus of adult attention.

For these autobiographers, the sound group for early childhood was the family, where music functioned to communicate a sense of mutuality and belonging. First memories were of singing, followed by dancing and playing; music making both reflected and produced family culture. There were patterns of development that reflected changes from childhood naiveté to more complex ideas of expertise and awareness of emulated models, accessed by increased exposure to a greater variety of ecologies, such as school music classes, private lessons, and independently chosen peer groups. In adolescence and young adulthood, individual stories of dispositional continuity and disruption were salient, often a factor of the interaction between competing ecologies or changes in those already existing. In this chapter, I focus specifically on early musical experiences with family members, where most musical memories are foundational and relational.

Family as Sound Group: Music, Ritual, and Spontaneity

In the Western world, childhood is a protected, naive time of life during which we acquire cultural knowledge and skills through both implicit and explicit means (Darian-Smith & Pascoe, 2013; Lum & Whiteman, 2012). Characterized by a natural curiosity and the drive to belong, it is a specific period of becoming, where learning is exponential and highly concentrated. It is also when we are particularly receptive to the foundational nature of human activity and the contexts in which that activity is experienced. In early childhood, it is the family as sound group that is at the center of most all the musical memories shared from that period. I am defining family as an individually conceptualized community including parents, siblings, grandparents, and any other people the participants chose to include under that umbrella.

Ecologies of Music at Home

In most of these autobiographies, music in early childhood is remembered as relationship-based activity, where dyadic and group affiliations were developed and nurtured. Music making contains the potential for both ritual and spontaneity—tradition and imagination working hand in hand. I begin with two snapshots of the musical lives of families involving dancing, singing, and instrument playing experiences. In the first, a weekly ritual is described, one that derives meaning from its anticipated outcome of spontaneous expression:[1]

> My musical history from birth through preschool was formed by my family. A memory of particular joy was visiting my maternal grandparents' home every Sunday for dinner. After dinner, Grandpa would gather all his grandchildren . . . and bring his guitar to sit on a very elaborate, curved chair. He would announce, "Get me my pick!" We would all scurry for it and in a few minutes, Grandpa would begin his dancing songs for us. I can't remember any particular tune just now, but I vividly recall dancing and laughing and always begging for more songs. (Deirdre, 1998)

The detail recalled here is in the visual memory ("the elaborate, curved chair") and the emotional encoding of the physical experience. This time together was a family ritual, remembered not for the repertoire, but for how it felt to engage together. The ritual provides a framework for anticipation and opportunity for expectations being realized, which is at the same time both comforting and generative.

A second snapshot is rich in sensory detail, not only visual depictions, but also sounds, rhythms of movement, and even smells. It, too, includes extended family members. The event is prompted by the actions of a young child, whose spontaneous playing initiates an immersive experience for a large group of elders:

> Later, we migrate into the living room, where we sit in a circle on velvet couches, forest green wooden chairs, Chippendale seats, and my abuela, like the Queen of Sheba, lands on the chocolate leather recliner. . . . Out of nowhere, a pint-sized cousin totters into the lively living room with a soup pot and a wooden spoon. This is the moment. My aunts dash and dive into the kitchen, opening the cabinets; the ruckus breaks out as they dig for the loudest, biggest, shiniest pots and pans they can find. They hand them out furiously to grasping, eager hands and I sprint to turn on the stereo.
>
> With Tito Puente blasting in the background, we cha-cha-cha to an insane steel drum solo. Those without spoons hit their pots with their hands,

---

[1] By ritual here, I am using Victor Turner's (1969) interpretation of ritual as a universal form of social action that unifies a group and can be re-created to maintain that unity.

and those without pots hit tops like cymbals. The dominó team can't resist the urge to join our party any longer, and they meet the dance, clanking dominoes together in their hands. Someone begins a conga line around the house and we snake through the den, through my brother's room, through the kitchen, through the family room. We go at it again and again, laughing and crashing into one another, like a school of fish changing shape in and out of currents.

My grandmother's skin smells clean from her Maja soap, my Aunt's damp with Cartier perfume, my mother's soft from her daily Nivea treatment. My cousin's dark, silky hair whizzes by me and I reach my arm out to stroke its brilliance, but she slips away from my fingers, falling into the center of the mass. I soon follow her, becoming lost in the essence.

Here, colliding with my relatives, I know who I am. I am not merely a number, an average grade, a statistic. I am not just a dutiful daughter, a loyal friend, a dedicated student. As raw as potatoes before we boil them for fricassee, my family allows me to be natural, pure. Returning to the palms of Cuba, the fig trees in Syria, the olive trees in Italy, I know where I am from, without boundaries or labels. I am these people, and I am their music. We are music. (Jacqueline, 2015)

The writer is recalling an experience ten years prior, at which time I believe she was in her early adolescence, and the clarity of her memory is astonishing. One can sense the fullness of the event and its meaning for her. The diversity of this group of aunts, grandmother (the Queen of Sheba), children, and domino players (presumably male relatives) conjures images of an open togetherness, with multiple responses contributing to the experience, each with integrity and purpose. Here, there is no hierarchy of expertise or preassigned role—all are encompassed in the whole and choose their mode of participation.

Music provides a ritual framework that draws individuals to the group and invites multiple entry points to relationship. In both examples, the experiences reflected familiarity in the people and musical practices involved, as well as novelty, in the opportunity for spontaneous response to the musical cues. This symbiosis creates ideal conditions for children's learning, where exploration and play lead to discovery, and where the agency afforded by possibilities to join the musical groups on their own volition is a powerful motivator.

FORMING RELATIONSHIPS   41

Family Music in Additional Spaces

Most of the autobiographical excerpts featured so far have taken place in the home. However, there were two settings where family music making occurred that were mentioned by multiple participants, offering specific characteristics that differed from home: religious institutions and the family car. In the first of these three examples, the rituals of music making in church supply material for both (spontaneous) imaginative play and skill development that shape home music life:

Example 1
There are home videos of my mother singing in the church choir while she was pregnant with me. The rhythms, sounds, and movements of the African American church experience have been the foundation of my musical exploration even at the pre-natal stage. . . . From infancy to toddler age of development, I have vivid memories of playing some type of percussive instrument whether it was a tambourine, shaker, African drums, or other household items that made noise. I was always intrigued by my surroundings and would find ways to re-create the plethora of sounds I experienced in church. I remember climbing on top of the kitchen cabinets at my home in New Jersey and pulling out pots/pans out of the cupboard. I would pretend the pan was a big tambourine and drum on top of the soup pot. Screams, hollers, and what I thought were sung sounds would follow these noises. My father was the choir director and lead musician at our church growing up so he would spend many hours rehearsing music for rehearsal and worship services at home. He would always watch me playing around the house and one Sunday morning he decided to put me on the drum set for the service. I was terrified, but I am thankful for the experience. Without it, I would not be self-taught on the set today. (Eric, 2016)

Example 2
Between first and second grade my family moved to . . . a town on the North Shore of Long Island. I joined a choral group at the reformed synagogue for children in the congregation. The group was . . . led by a soft-spoken, maternal cantor. Once a week, I would go to the temple and learn Hebrew songs and Jewish songs in English with friends. One of the highlights of this experience was performing during the children's services for the High Holy

Days. The songs taught me about Jewish culture, probably even more than my experiences in Hebrew school, and the music connected me to yet another community. (Hillary, 2004)

Example 3
Growing up in church also had a significant influence on me. The first time I ever got goose bumps while listening to a piece of music was when singing "I Know Who Holds Tomorrow" with Grandpa at a church service. I might be too young at the time to appreciate the music itself, but the emotions accompanied by the song and by the expressions on people's faces while singing the song completely touched me. In addition, singing Christmas carols was one of my favorite activities of the year. We lit candles and stood in front of crowded stores to spread the gospel. Later in life I continued to serve in church and although I never considered myself religious, hymns had touched me more often than any other genres of music. (Fanny, 2004)

In considering the church-home mesosystem (Bronfenbrenner's name for the interactions between two microsystems), we can see how it is the child strives to integrate multiple experiences using music as the vehicle to traverse settings. These early mixtures of neighboring communities into home life are among the first ways we begin defining ourselves.

Experiences recalled in the family car were ecologically defined: this setting is a confined space, keeping people (on occasion, involuntarily) together, often for long periods of time. Koops (2014) did a study of preschool (aged 10 months to 4.5 years) students enrolled in a family music class and tracked their use of songs in the car. She found that the repertoire materials were the same as were used at home; the family subculture supported the use of the same songs across different settings. Additionally, the physical proximity to siblings and the lack of distractions were enabling conditions for family music making in the car. The autobiographers in this sample had positive memories of music sharing during these rides, and the music, unlike in Koops's study, was more exclusive to the setting, in other words, songs specific to the car environment. Here are two examples:

Example 1
Riding in the car we had a special tape [my father] would put on and my favorite songs to sing with him were "Sweet Georgia Brown" and "Don't Get Around Much Anymore." He still has the record. My mother and I also sang in

the car on trips to Grandma's house in upstate New York. We sang the general car songs as well as *West Side Story, Barbra Streisand*, and when I was lucky, maybe one of my tapes like Huey Lewis and the News. We had a special Huey Lewis song called "Happy to Be Stuck with You" that seemed very appropriate for our situation. (Sarah, 2014)

Example 2
Our family often took long drives in the car to West Malaysia (north of Singapore) during holidays such as the Lunar New Year. As usual, I would sit on my own in the backseat of the car but keeping myself entertained by looking out of window, asking questions occasionally, listening to my parents' conversations, and listening to the radio. I clearly remember the festive Mandarin songs over the radio broadcast during our Lunar New Year road trips—the loud jolly tunes, male and female duets, drums and cymbals. (Sirene, 2005)

Recollections of singing in the car were less frequent in the more recently collected autobiographies. I surmise that the advent of specially targeted technological innovation, with its ability to individualize entertainment options, has resulted in changes in the ways families interact in this setting.

Family members were key players in these more public settings—singing favorite songs with a father or listening to a mother sing in church. In this next section, I include stories shared about specific family relationships, demonstrating the patterns and diversities among memories, and positing the psychological and sociological influences that guide our remembering.

Music and Family Member Roles: Learning to Be Together

Mothers and Fathers: Comforters, Companions, Disc Jockeys, Teachers

As mentioned earlier, music making in family contexts is primarily about securing relationships (Malloch & Trevarthen, 2009). Interactions with parents are the most prevalent experiences described in the early childhood portions of these autobiographies. Memories indicate that they engaged in musical conversations, sang in order to comfort, performed for and with infants, and introduced children to musical repertoire. The association of specific music with parents can be so strong as to create a feeling of their presence, even when they are physically absent"

> *My parents are not musicians and did not listen to a lot of music. However, at home they had a record I remember very well. It was a Teresa Brewer album, and the song I loved was, "Music! Music! Music!" I remember holding the album cover, knowing it was something belonging to my parents. Playing the music they loved, even if they were not around, was perhaps a way to connect with them. (Hillary, 2004)*

Here, the album cover serves as a transitional object (Winnecott, 1971), providing a way to bring the comforting parental presence to mind when they are physically absent. In many of the autobiographies, writers could conjure specific moments in time with family members; beyond physical artifacts, engagement in musical activity can serve as what Pigrum (2009) might refer to as a transitional practice. Through practices of listening to and performing music we build futures shaped by associations with our past. Accrued memories can serve as resources to be accessed for comfort, expression, and communication.

Thinking back to the links between memory and positive emotion, it is no surprise that an image and the concomitant sound could conjure such a deep connection. These musical connections start even before birth, as some participants found in interviewing their parents, and I continue with a brief review of early memories of infancy, which often are parental memories passed along rather than explicit memories of the writers. I also look at possible differences between mothers and fathers, and how the music our parents share with us become part of our own repertoire, informing our cultural identities.

Another mechanism for connecting is the reciprocal interaction of communicative musicality (Custodero, 2009), in which the parent and infant engage in conversation structured by a shared pulse and narrative form (Malloch & Trevarthen, 2009). These proto-conversations are a result of a desire for mutuality—to see oneself in another—and to sense belonging (to a sound group). Below, a writer recounts her surprise discovery of a treasure that provides evidence of this:

> *I was exposed to singing as an infant, when my mother would cradle me in her arms while singing traditional Korean children's songs. But there is one*

particular incident that stands out and was recorded on a tape by my father. As an adolescent, I came across this tape of my dad and I having a musical conversation when I was a toddler. In this recording, my dad would sing a line of a Korean pop song and I would respond with my own musical humming and noises. It was amazing listening to this tape for the first time because in this tape, I was obviously at an age where I was not yet able to speak. But my ability as a young child to communicate with my father in a musical way was fascinating. (Shirley, 2004)

In the new millennium, documenting children's early music making in photographs, audio, and video has become a way to preserve memories and shape the ways we remember. These representations of life events are accessible to be reviewed an infinite number of times; even so, our memories of the event may change over time because our life experiences change the way we view ourselves. The discovery of such artifacts provides new information about oneself and a direct link to the perspective and values of the person doing the recording.

Not surprisingly, the most cited family member is the mother: 75 percent of the student autobiographies include specific references to musical interactions with her. Recollections of intimate music making with mothers were common. Typically, these experiences were remembered as calming and personal. Below, repertoire mingles with feeling to reconstruct the memory:

My earliest musical experience is hearing a lullaby that my mother wrote for me. She wrote one for all her children, but I always thought mine was the most personal. She would sing "Daddy's in the other room, both your brothers are asleep. Once again tonight it seems, it's just Kirky Lynne and me. So dream your little dreams, smile your little smiles. Let your mama hold you close for just a little while...." I remember hearing my mom's voice sing the lullaby, and that's the only time I would ever hear her sing. (Kirstin, 2004)

We can almost hear the softness of the mother's voice, delivering the intimate lyric: this excerpt suggests a social bonding between child and mother. It is sanctified time, set apart from the rest of the day vis-à-vis its musical character, and set apart from the rest of the family in a particular place.

Singing is a way in which both mothers and fathers bond with their children; however, some research involving lullaby singing indicates that parents are more expressive with same-sex infants (Trehub et al., 1997).[2] There was a sense that mutuality for mothers and daughters was heightened in some instances, as suggested by the excerpt above: *"Daddy's in the other room, both your brothers are asleep. Once again tonight it seems, it's just Kirky Lynne and me."* As described by Lawler (2000), this can be interpreted as a "Mothering of Self" and extends into a female child's future maternal experiences. The following excerpt alludes to the depth of this connection:

My very first musical learning started so early that I do not even remember. My first teacher was my mother who was a fine singer. When I was young, she sang to me various songs such as children's songs, Korean folk songs, and arias, and then led me to sing after her. She sang really softly and warmly so I could sense her love. She told me after my baby was born that she started singing to me right after my birth and I began to sing after her when I was eighteen months old. When I stayed with my parents after my daughter's birth, we (me and my mother) had a chance to sing together the "songs of ours" to my daughter, which tied all three of us together. I hope to share the same love for music with my daughter that I shared with my mother. (Su-Young, 2004)

Fathers were mentioned in close to half of the autobiographies collected and had their own roles in the family music making that often complemented the mother's role. In the following excerpt, the specific contributions of each parent are clear:

One of my earliest musical memories involves my mother singing me to sleep. While I do not remember the words to most of the songs she would sing, I do remember the soothing, calming, quality of her voice. Her singing worked to make me feel safe, loved, and completely content as I drifted off to sleep.

My father, on the other hand, who identifies himself as tone-deaf, would only sing to me in contexts where his singing could be viewed as a joke. He would make up songs about how it was time to get shoes on, time for bed, or time to eat breakfast. His songs brought joy to everyday tasks and taught me how to recognize the fun in music. While I enjoyed his songs, I never asked my father to sing me to sleep because I always felt that my mother was better suited for the job. Mom's songs put me to sleep, Dad's songs made me laugh.

---

[2] Such a perspective must be approached with a great deal of caution, especially in light of the changing roles of women in the workplace, and the diversity demonstrated in contemporary cross-cultural research on fatherhood (e.g., Roopnarine, 2015).

Both of my parents do not consider themselves to be musicians, and yet it's their constant use of song in the household that provided me with some of my earliest exposures to music. (Kelly, 2015)

It was common for parental roles to be different; however, the roles weren't necessarily gendered or consistent across stories. What remained constant was the use of music to connect with one another:

Before I was born and especially in my first few months after birth, my mother took care to play various recordings of the Bach cello suites for me. From that same time through [my] first few years, both parents sang many nursery rhymes, lullabies and folk songs to and with me—mostly in French, as a common bond for us all, since my father is from France and my mother from Canada. This was a way for them to connect and also include my grandparents in my upbringing. My father in particular has a singing voice that I find soothing and comforting to this day. I can imagine it in my head without actually hearing the voice live. (Matt, 2016)

Here, the mother and father play different roles. The male writer of this excerpt comments on memories of his father's singing, providing a counter narrative to the stereotypical image of father as distant observer or rough-and-tumble playmate.

Relationships are generated and sustained through sharing what is meaningful and communicating vulnerability as we reveal what we love to a child. I believe we do this because they trust us to care for them, and we, in turn, learn to trust them to enjoy what we enjoy. One student wrote about how her father loved a specific musician, and about how that love taught her about her dad:

My childhood is full of memories of listening to music both in my family's home and at concerts. My dad considers it one of his biggest regrets that he never took me to see the Grateful Dead, but after all, I was only seven when Jerry Garcia passed away. The day that he died is a powerful memory for me because it's when I truly came to understand how much my father loved Jerry. It was as Sunday morning and my dad was driving me home from Hebrew School. . . . As we pulled into our garage, my mom was standing in the entryway to the house, and I could tell by her posture and the tears in her eyes that something was wrong. As my dad and I got out of his Land Cruiser (of

> course, plastered in Grateful Dead bears, skulls, and roses), my mom looked at my dad and said, "Jerry died." My dad chucked his bag . . . across the garage, retreated into his room and didn't retreat from it for two whole days. I think of this day often when I consider the musicians I loved. I admire and enjoy listening to many artists, but there isn't one artist who has had such a profound effect on my life that I would have a reaction as strong as my father's if they passed away. Some may call his reaction the result of fanaticism or obsession—and maybe it is, but my dad's deep love for Jerry undoubtedly added meaning and beauty to his life—like any great love does. Over this past weekend, we shared a teary hug at the conclusion of the Dead's Fare Thee Well concert that we watched on pay-per-view. It was a striking moment for me. I was surprised at how emotional I got. After all, the Grateful Dead had always been my dad's passion, not necessarily mine. Like we talked about in class yesterday, it really hit me how the music we identify with becomes a huge part of our identities. To love my father isn't to love the Grateful Dead, but to love my father is to love that HE loves the Grateful Dead. (Elise, 2015)

Grandparents: Champions and Playmates

According to Pilkauskas and Martinson (2014), over a quarter of US children in the early childhood range live in three-generation households. Interestingly, after mothers and fathers, memories of early childhood musical experiences with grandparents were mentioned most often (27%). They were typically different from interactions with parents, often more tolerant:

> The first musical memory I have comes from when my maternal grandparents took me to church with them when I was two years old. Though the details remain rather fuzzy as I reflect back on them now, I can recall sitting in between Grandpa and Grandma Muzzy and listening to everyone singing the processional hymn. I was fascinated! My eyes grew wide with enchantment as I took in the sounds of the organ in harmony with the voices of the people around me. When the hymn was over and everyone sat down, I decided it was my turn to sing, and so I chose the only tune I knew: "A, B, C, D, E, F, G!" I burst out from the bench, smiling and wiggling my legs back and forth. I was so filled with excitement about this musical cultural activity that I just had to join in. My grandparents turned and looked at me with delight as I continued. Soon the pastor and the other churchgoers turned and smiled

at this pleasant interruption to their Sunday morning service. This was but the beginning of what I hope to be a lifelong relationship to music and music making. (Joanna, 2016)

Grandmothers were remembered as adults who served needs that arose in childhood—sometimes first piano teachers and sometimes playmates, as in this excerpt:

Whenever I visited my grandma . . . I would always ask her to play the Cabbage Patch or Strawberry Shortcake records. We would listen to them while drawing pictures and making crafts. She also had a record in German that had traditional songs; one of these songs was called "Erika." You can only imagine how much this excited me. I would march around the house to the beat of the music, as if I was in a marching band. (Erika, 2004)

In many autobiographies, grandfathers were seen as characters larger than life (recall the first sound group example). Just as fathers have taken on more child-rearing responsibilities in the last fifty years, grandfathers are becoming more actively involved in the lives of grandchildren (Buchanan & Rotkirch, 2016). This rather long but telling excerpt shows the impact one family member can have:

A big influence in my musical development since my early childhood . . . [was] my late grandfather. He had a great impact on my general development and was a very important figure in my life. He was a singer, and also played the guitar. . . . However, he was also a great Byzantine chanter in church and also sang traditional Greek music in local fiestas. I grew up with him, he was always next to me and out of six children and thirteen grandchildren I was his favorite, which also balanced my middle child insecure syndrome. Music was part of him, he would sing very often it seemed almost all the time; he would hum a melody when working, in his quiet moments, when drinking coffee or just sitting under the trees, he would sing out loud and even dance on his own melodies. But mostly he loved singing along with us, the children, he would teach us different songs and improvise funny story telling songs to make us laugh. He was full of music but in a very natural way; he was not trying to be musical or integrate music in his life, it seemed to him that naturally everything was musical. Spending a lot of time during my childhood with such a musically creative person had a major impact in my musical life. In a very

> *nurturing and loving environment I learned how to listen and embrace music; I primarily learned how to listen to the music of nature and the music inside me. I am not sure how to explain it but through this informal educational encounter I learned the most important musical lessons; I discovered and felt the wholeness of music, a feeling that balanced many conflicting questions inside me. (Lina, 2004)*

Here, a grandfather provides a model of "musical living," which, experienced in childhood, shaped the direction and character of a musician-educator. In the next excerpt, there is a sense of affiliation with no memory. But just as we reconstruct our memories to fit the circumstances of the retelling, we can imagine encounters of mutuality—of seeing oneself in another—that exceed the boundaries of mortality.

> *One thing that in the recent years that has been important to me musically was finding a recording of my grandfather's band. My grandfather was a New York City circuit-wedding musician that worked on weekends. He played accordion. Sadly, he passed away when I was around one year old. I never got to know him but my family members always compared me to him saying I was the musician in the family from him. My father didn't have any recordings of him so my whole life I always wanted to hear how he sounded. One day in 2007, I Googled his name and I found that the son of the bass player from their wedding band posted ten recordings of the band from their gigs and demos. This was an amazing find and was amazing to hear. He even played some of the same songs that I learned in recent years. It was a pleasure for our whole family to have recordings of this band and these recordings are special to me because after twenty years, I was able to hear his band play. (Christian, 2012)*

In these two examples, both involving grandfathers, we see the strong need for heritage and how that need generates relationships that go beyond physical presence.

Siblings: Allies and Partners in Pretend

The last family group I will consider in this section is siblings. Interactions with siblings are unlike those involving parents or grandparents because they come directly from other children. The imaginative play and imitation of adult behaviors common in children's play (Singer & Singer, 1990) characterize stories of musical play as well.

> *On April 21, 1998, my little brother, Albert, was born and I voluntarily took on the responsibility of sharing our family's musical repertoire with him. At night, I was still a recipient of lullabies, but I also joined my parents in serenading Albert to sleep. Eventually, when Albert was older, we sang lullabies to our stuffed animals in play-pretend games, like "house." Later in life, we branched out to other genres, and performed together for our family around the holidays. (Francesca, 2017)*

Family culture is both extended and expanded by the play of siblings. There is a shared history of the home environment that finds its way to the imaginative play described above and provides a way to cope with the struggles of childhood, as is evident in this excerpt:

> *I can remember myself in preschool choreographing duets with my sister, mostly on classical music, according to my mother our favorite was Dvořák Symphony No. 7; we would create a play, sort of a ballet and sometimes we would use dolls for the characters that were missing. Later on, my youngest sister would play all the extra roles. I remember making costumes from clothes around the house and announcing to our parents the official performance/show. Sometimes the plot of our ballet would be a caricature of our parents' behavior and incidents of our everyday life; I can see now we creatively and very cleverly criticized them while at the same time we expressed ourselves through music and dance, and they could only applaud us and maybe awkwardly smile! These musical activities gave us a great sense of freedom: a creative freedom of expression, communication and self-discovery. (Lina, 2004)*

As in the example above, this final excerpt demonstrates the abandon with which siblings and friends might engage in imaginative play, here reaping aesthetic rewards through the embodiment of musical icons:

> *My family lived in Merrick, Long Island, on a cul-de-sac street with several other children. Another memory from this period involves Jeffrey and Jordan, two boys on the block who were about the same age as me and my sister [sic]. We used to be two sets of Donny and Marie, singing the songs from the TV*

show into battery-operated microphones, and hairbrushes when we broke the microphones. (Hillary, 2004)

This musical play with siblings is part of child culture, taking on the qualities of peer group play that is purposeful and imitative of the surroundings. It exists separately from adult culture and is differentiated in content and context.

Our musical interactions with family members have lasting consequences, as they remain in our present consciousness as memories retold and reimagined by others and ourselves. Engaging in child-initiated play with siblings, connecting to a multigenerational heritage with grandparents, and learning how to be with others through parents serving as "musical companions" inculcate children into the social world. They also function as cultural gatekeepers for this early period through sharing their own preferences and values manifested in the activities they share.

Music in Neighborhood and Societal Contexts

Whether through French folk songs, rock 'n' roll, or Teresa Brewer's "Music, Music, Music!," parents inculcate in their children a world of specific repertoire styles and practices. Parental preferences shape our musical lives, and because they are delivered in the context of relationship, they are deeply connected to our sense of self.

My earliest recollection of music is my mother singing and dancing with me in her arms to the Frank Sinatra version of Irving Berlin's "Cheek to Cheek." . . . This was not a strange occurrence in Brooklyn that an African American mother in the mid-60s was dancing and singing around her small apartment with her infant son, her first child, listening to an Italian American from New Jersey singing a song from a Jewish American from New York. It was simply eclectic. This is my life and where I found my love for music in very humble beginnings. (Leonard, 2004)

Eclecticism was prominent in many autobiographies, especially those written by people like the writer of the previous excerpt, who grew up in New York City, where access to diverse music practices characterizes residential life.

In contrast, there are stories of people from homogeneous societies whose early musical experience was defined by an enlarged sense of a singular national culture:

> *Singing and music flow through my veins! My earliest recollection of growing up in Wales is of being surrounded by music. Even the mountains sing! Wales is traditionally known as "the land of the song," and "to be born Welsh is to be born with music in your blood and poetry in your soul" (a Welsh proverb). How blessed I am to have grown up there. For some reason, when I think back on my childhood days, the song ["Sospan Fach"] always comes to mind. I'm not quite sure why exactly, but that's the beauty of folk songs. They exist, passing down from generation to generation, often orally until they are so ingrained in a tradition that no explanation is needed. This particular song is sung whenever a group of Welsh people gathers together—in primary schools; in "eisteddfodau" [music and poetry festivals]; during rugby games (especially when the Welsh play England!); in a "Gymanfa Ganu" (where people travel to a designated church and have a hymn-singing festival); in pubs; and yes, it has been known to have been sung during a funeral! (Peris, 2004)*

It is interesting to consider how the same music can be malleable to changes in settings. That it can have meaning at a rugby game and a funeral implies that the ecological context confers the meaning, rather than the music, which serves multiple functions vis-à-vis its identification with the general public. Representing the familiar and the collective, the folk song can express grief, celebration, camaraderie, and religious verve. This contrasts with the first example, where a specific piece of music was purposefully used to establish an intimate relational context.

Infants and young children are enculturated into music both directly, in those intimate settings of the home with parents, and indirectly, through the larger societies in which their parents exist. The intersections of public media culture and local personal culture are sometimes at odds. One of the most notable examples in recent history was the media coverage of the "Mozart Effect." Because I was an academic researcher involved with the Grammy Foundation's collaborative project with Mead Johnson, which produced two classical music CDs for new mothers, I was uniquely positioned to witness this intersection. One afternoon in 1999, I received a desperate phone call from a new mother. She was concerned that her husband might be doing something to disadvantage their new daughter. When I asked what he was doing, she replied that he was dancing with her in his arms and singing to her with music by the iconic soul man, James Brown. She was a college professor, and I assume wanted to give her first child every possible opportunity to maximize the potential for her future. I share this to demonstrate the power of popular culture to influence parenting, in this case for at least a decade, beginning in the mid-1990s. The claims that classical music is better for babies than other music parents love (such as James Brown) was an extrapolation at best: research literature showing Mozart's music improved spatial-temporal reasoning was done with college students, and not infants (Rausher et al., 1993).

I also share this story because several of the autobiographies suggested this issue was an influence, as in this next excerpt. The student here is a product of her time, clearly influenced by the 2004 zeitgeist, when the Mozart Effect research was being interpreted and marketed as a "parenting guide":

My mother always reminisces about how much classical music she played for me while she was pregnant with me and when I was a young child. She said that Mozart was always heard around the house; so much that she even became "sick of it." However, she knew that exposing me to that music at such an early age would have a positive impact on my musical and mental development. To this day, she (and I) credit my initial inclination towards music on her decision to immerse me as a child in classical music. I suppose I can say that my musical life began even before I was born! (Theresa, 2004)

It should also be noted that in a national survey administered in 2000 (Custodero, Britto, & Xin, 2002; Custodero & Johnson-Green, 2003; Custodero & Johnson-Green, 2008), the Parents Use of Music with Infants Study, we found that parents were much more likely to use music with their infants for social-emotional reasons than to make their children smarter, despite the popular media representation of classical music as having privileged status.

Memories of family music making were expressed far more often in the autobiographies than interactions consciously intended as investment in future outcomes. However, the immediate rewards of musical engagement, intuitively enacted, had long-term effects on the participants through the repeated iterations that were used to construct their musical self-image.

Constructing a Musical Self through Relationships

We are each an amalgam of our past, present, and future. Autobiographical memories of our earliest years provide windows through which we can examine how our past still lives in our present, to have a sense of ourselves as complete historical beings with promise for continued growth. Looking from the inside out, we can see the self and self-other constructions (Gulbrandsen, 2012) that have been in development since childhood. We draw from our past experiences to situate ourselves in the immediate and varied circumstances of our roles as student, musician, family member, and teacher in a continuous process of recollection and reflection.

Our childhoods provide stories that eventually become our own personal heritage. This chapter's focus has been on the ecological spaces and interactive social contexts in which we first experience music, and the meaning of these memories for our current artistic selves. Those of us who have strong explicit memories of music making can access them as a way of defining our current selves, as did the author of the richly descriptive sound group example: "I know where I am from, without boundaries or labels. I am these people, and I am their music. We are music." The emotional response to musical participation with those she loved created an expansive sense of unity. Damasio (2010) reminds us that the autobiographical self includes all social phenomena, including the "social self" and the "spiritual self" (p. 23). To conclude, I review the memories of interactive musical experiences in childhoods as they are positioned in familial place, relationship and heritage.

The Ecologies of Early Music Experiences: "I Know Where I Am From"

In most all the examined memories from early childhood, *where* I am from was commensurate with *who* I am from. The "place" of musical activity was situated in the family unit. In other words, place was delineated by people rather than institutional, architectural, or geographical boundaries. How were these family units constituted? The definitions were varied, ranging from reports of intimately sung lullabies by one parent to a child, to a host of relations dancing and playing makeshift instruments in a conga line. A national population is conceived of as family through its common musical experience of a folk song: *"This particular song is sung whenever a group of Welsh people gathers together."*

The recalled experiences most often occurred in a home of the immediate family, or that of a grandparent or extended family member, although most of the time it was not explicitly stated but was intimated by the activity description. Only about 20 percent of the autobiographies mentioned a specific locale (e.g., city or country) associated with their early years; still, naming their place was in addition to, not in lieu of, naming family members. One notable exception was again the story from Wales, where life was situated in landscape: *"Singing and music flows through my veins! My earliest recollection of growing up in Wales is of being surrounded by music. Even the mountains sing!"*

The two settings other than home that were named in the stories confirm this permeating role of family as place: the car had meaning because memories are of specific repertoire shared with family members in a bounded space; the church or synagogue provided an extended family who took on musically supportive roles. Instrumental and vocal ensembles provided possibilities to engage in performance, prompting memories of skill development. Memories of congregations participating in spiritually communal singing provoked feelings reminiscent of the intense responses found in recollections of strong experiences in music (Gabrielsson, 2011). As one excerpt offered, *"the emotions accompanied by the song and by the expressions on people's faces while singing the song completely touched me."*

Feeling "touched" represents a link, a connection to what unites us as humans. One of the quoted excerpts reads, *"I have especially vivid memories of this music, because it evokes memories at a time when my family was together, singing together."* The musical interactions with family members took many forms: singing, moving/dancing, playing instruments, listening to music; musical encounters were experienced as "being with" both person(s) and musical sound (Custodero, 2005).

Being Together in Harmony: "I Am These People, and I Am Their Music"

The social nature of the musical experience served to strengthen relationships through creating conditions that cultivate expressivity, communication, and comfort.

Psychologists have conceptualized many theories about how and when our social lives develop, starting in infancy and continuing throughout the lifespan. Examples include looking at how a baby becomes *attached* to a caregiver (Bowlby, 1982), suggesting a physical joining; how interacting with a *transitional object* (Winnecott, 1971) serves as an associative substitute for a parent physically absent from the setting; and how parents learn to read and match their children's emotional states, offering support through *affect attunement* (Stern, 1985, 2010).

The notions of attachment, association, and attunement are exemplified in the autobiographical stories here; that is, they affirm the permeating recollections of relationship. Parental singing and music listening routines made participants feel comforted and "safe" (securely attached). Later, the same repertoire could be accessed, even by adults, as a (transitional) object associated with those subjective feelings around family music making. These songs and pieces may also be shared with one another in a process of affect attunement, which involves sympathetic attempts to be with, to deeply know that person. Turino (2008) describes this phenomenon in particularly gratifying music making contexts of adults, "where the identification with others is so direct and so intense that we feel . . . as if our selves had merged" (p. 19).

Coming into relationship is how culture is acquired. As was mentioned earlier, Dissanayake (2000) uses the term *mutuality* to address the psychobiological need to see oneself in another; it is the discovery of kinship. Consider the story of the woman who had the chance to hear a tape of herself as an infant, responding musically to her father's singing a Korean pop song. She was surprised at what she called her *"ability as a young child to communicate . . . in a musical way."* This artifact provided experiences in two spheres of mutuality: one, her father's inculcating her into the mutual understanding of what a song means; and two, her own sense of ontological mutuality—to recognize her adult self in this documentation of her infant self and to have an experience of coherence. The seven-year-old watching the final Grateful Dead concert with her father experienced a similar epiphany: *"It was a striking moment for me. I was surprised at how emotional I got."* Later in demonstration of sympathetic understanding, she writes *"to love my father is to love that HE loves the Grateful Dead."*

Our childhoods are spent in a constant state of enculturation—learning how to belong with the people in our environments. Music experiences connect us to people with a sense of belonging, merging with them to become an attuned entity, responding to the needs of the present moment. In our earliest interactions, we seek to join as a way of learning how to be in the world. Later, as we gain awareness of ourselves as separate beings, we seek to join as a complement to others, basking in the delight of coming together in new ways, invoking imitation and variation. I witnessed one of the most beautiful examples of this symbiosis at a concert in South Africa in 1998. It was a collaborative project involving two seemingly disparate sound groups: I Fagiolini, a Renaissance choral group from Oxford, and the SDASA Chorale from Soweto. They shared in each other's songs, each maintaining the integrity of their own sound traditions, resulting in a formerly unimaginable performance. Pieces included a Zulu chant joined with an early sixteenth-century English song, and a contrapuntal Agnus Dei woven into a Xhosa harmonic pattern. The project was called "Simunye," a Zulu word translating to "we are one."

Receiving and Creating Musical Heritage: "I Know Who I Am"

As children, we are both recipients and creators of musical heritage—inducted into musical practices by family and community while also influencing those practices as they are experienced anew. As we grow into adulthood, we often have a yearning to share a heritage—it is a way to bring our own past to the present and take it into the future through passing it on. Many examples in this chapter reflect such synergy: the story of a mother, grateful for her own mother's song and looking forward to sharing it with her child; a father's immense love for Jerry Garcia, shared and accepted; and the overwhelming need of a fellow musician to hear what a grandfather's accordion playing sounded like, even though he was no longer living.

A few of the autobiographies contained particularly powerful examples of how memories of meaningful childhood experiences became resources for adult lives:

> *Spending a lot of time during my childhood with [my grandfather who was] such a musically creative person had a major impact in my musical life. In a very nurturing and loving environment I learned how to listen and embrace music; I primarily learned how to listen to the music of nature and the music inside me. (Lina, 2004)*

And when the music repertoire takes on associations with feelings, the sharing is especially poignant, as those feelings become associated with the people involved. Associations with childhood music making can become part of our identity and keep us whole, they serve to keep us mindful of the comfort, safety, and freedom many of us experience in those years.

Retrieving musical memories from our early years can bring surprise, affirmation, confusion, and feelings of missed opportunity. Through reflecting on our past, we can better understand the present, now informed by the experiences that preceded our current roles and actions. We also can shape the future from a more informed stance, taking "I know who I am" to "I know who I want to be."

4
A Sense of Musical Self

Engaging Dispositions and Claiming Identities

Conceptualizing Musical Selves

My family had a hammock made of rope set up in the backyard. I have a distinct memory of swinging on the hammock, looking at the sky through the trees and singing, "This Land Is Your Land." I believe I associated the lyrics with the natural surroundings. This is a memory that evokes an emotion of being alone, yet feeling at peace, comforted by nature. Around kindergarten, I have a very strong memory of announcing to my family and friends that my favorite song was "You Are the Woman That I Always Dreamed Of." I think that the song was by the band Firefly. Perhaps this announcement was a way of establishing individuality. I had a sense of certainty about how the music affected me. The music seemed to help me understand and articulate my sense of self. (Hillary, 2004)

Music preferences and participation provide means by which we define ourselves. This sense of self changes over time, due to the increased consciousness of our increasingly varied environments and the perceived possibilities of engagement. In this excerpt, Hillary mentions two memories of experiences with specific songs, one in which she feels joined to the natural world, blurring the distinction between self and environment into a type of peaceful solitude; and another she considers "a way of establishing individuality," distinguishing herself as a separate entity with her own predilections. It is the internal negotiating of those two circumstances, fitting in and standing out, that shapes us as musicians, and music's capacity for offering both collective experience and individual expression—exerting our own sense of rightness as well as "losing ourselves" in an act of participation (Frith, 1996)—that shapes our humanity.

In the previous chapter we looked at the earliest memories of music education students, which were centered on feelings, mainly generated by our

Before We Teach Music. Lori A. Custodero, Oxford University Press. © Oxford University Press 2024.
DOI: 10.1093/oso/9780197557877.003.0004

interactions with family members. Participant stories reflected our roles as what McAdams (2015) calls Social Actors, advantaging our environments and the people in them, to answer fundamental questions about being in this world. At this first level, we are most conscious of the present—we find delight in discovery and novelty. By the age of two or three we display observable behavior, grounded in dispositions that carry messages about *how* we do music, referred to as "know how" by Damasio (1999, p. 139). By middle childhood, those messages show some consistency and interact with dynamic experiences and stable personality traits to contribute to the perception of identities, signaling who we are as musicians—what McAdams refers to as Motivated Agents, a second level, with the capacity for linking present experiences to future possibilities. It is in McAdams's third developmental level beginning in mid-to-late adolescence that we begin looking at our past, using it to make sense of who we are through constructing historical narratives. As Autobiographical Authors, we take these stories into adulthood, composing a life that brings together past memories, the present moment and the anticipated future.

What do our childhood memories tell us about the ways in which we see our musical selves today? What moments hold meaning for us as we construct our musical life stories? In this chapter I explore music as dispositional knowledge, implicitly experienced by Social Actors and Motivated Agents, who are compelled to engage through the culturally familiar sounds and structures of the music. When recollected by Autobiographical Authors, these stories become an explicit way of understanding our musical selves. Later, I address mechanisms of response to music and to music education practices using the lens of dispositional personality traits (McAdams, 2015), tracing how these aspects of self are activated in various musical contexts. Following this focus on the individual experience, I discuss how identity is constructed through encounters with musical instruments and musical people and explore the ways in which exposure, access, and enculturation figure prominently in developmental pathways and the construction of musical identity.

Dispositions and the Power of Implicit Knowing

Middle childhood, a period roughly between the ages of seven and fourteen, was a time when many of these autobiographers recalled experiences critical to the formation of musical identities. These years often involved the onset of more formal music participation, and memories of epiphanies, challenges, and relationships with teachers and peers were shared. The musical self was constructed through the intersections of dispositions, opportunities, and environmental support systems. Looking through the multidisciplinary kaleidoscope, I examine dispositions from several lenses, including Neuroscience, Embodied Cognition, Human Development, and Social Psychology.

Implicit Musicality

Infants have what Trehub (2001) calls "predispositions" for music, demonstrated by their ability to process pitch contours and rhythmic patterns in much the same ways adults do—before they are explicitly utilized. She purports that music is a tool for adaptation, and that our musicality has evolved to meet psychological needs, first introduced through the vocal musical interactions between parent and child. If we are predisposed to construct meaning from musical experience, it follows that we have neural structures for managing dispositions for musical knowledge.

Neuroscientist Antonio Damasio describes dispositional knowledge as implicit—not representational like words or images, but innate unconscious knowing—or what he calls "abstract records of potentialities" (2010, p. 144). These are memories we cannot access directly until they become explicitly encoded into words or actions. Implicit knowledge precedes explicit knowledge and the enactment of rules and conscious thought: all words and images began as dispositions—as feelings we couldn't name. Two neural systems that Damasio calls "spaces" work to retrieve our implicit and explicit memories and are located in discrete regions interspersed throughout the brain. The *image* space constructs explicit maps of past musical experience; it does so from an aggregate of the early sensory cortices, the regions of the cerebral cortex located in and around sensory (e.g., visual and auditory) entry points to the brain. The *dispositional* space is found in the areas of the cortex not in use by the image space and involves higher-order associations vis-à-vis implicit knowing and its potential for reconstructing that knowledge through recall. Important to our context is that this implicit way of knowing is also responsible for generating movement. These two spaces work together to make sense of what we have experienced. This integrated structure of spaces is important to our examination of the musical self—it unites implicit and explicit thinking, as well as past, present, and potential (future) experience.

In many of the autobiographies there was mention of this dispositional musicality in the abilities discovered in childhood, often around playing "by ear." The satisfaction that rose up from those experiences was motivating, as can be seen in this excerpt from Jessica, who, when she was a master's student, called herself a "Cello Evangelist":

When I was ten, I decided I wanted to learn a new instrument. My dad hoped I would learn guitar like him, but I didn't want to get calluses and have to keep cutting my fingernails. Even though it didn't fit my instrument criteria, we had had a cello in the house for years and I wanted to give it a try. My mother got the cello for $70 thinking she would take lessons one day and I'd seen it in the house before, but the strings were always loose and unplayable. We took it to the living room; my dad strung it up and tried it a little first before giving it to me. I played the open strings and noticed a familiar tune between them. Then I plunked out "Habanera" from Carmen and became a cellist. (Jessica, 2000)

Her memory of this ability to "plunk out" a tune on an instrument she was experiencing for the first time suggests she may have a disposition for that particular way of making music. Characteristics in her genetic code and physicality to which she is biologically disposed joined with her past experience to create the "abstract record of potentiality" that facilitated this clarifying moment.

Singers also shared experiences of dispositional knowing. Memories of what marked the early stages of engagement for them involved active performance:

Lining my dolls along the windowsill of my bedroom as a five-year-old, teaching them the songs I felt they had to know from The Sound of Music, *was the beginning of my desire to become a musician. Hearing the lyrical voice of Julie Andrews play over and over again sparked my interest in singing, and I knew that I would one day perform on stage. For as far back as I can recall, my passion has been to sing. Whether I have been gazing across the Huang Pu River in Shanghai, China, or chugging along in an auto rickshaw through the crowded alleys of Hyderabad, India, a melody has constantly run through my head. As a child, I can remember dancing to the vibrant music of Miriam Makeba and Joan Baez in my grandparent's home in Hyderabad. The intricate melodies and beautiful phrases provided me with a sense of pulse and rhythm that [seemed to be] inherent. (Noor, 2013)*

Dispositional knowledge is relational. Our past takes on meaning as our memories help define our present; in terms of musical identity, we look at these moments of wonder (*"dancing to the vibrant music of Miriam Makeba"*) as mileposts on the journey to becoming our current musical selves. This wonder often leads to realizations of surprise achievement (Cobb, 1977), experienced in a momentary synthesis of disposition and potential, giving rise to a new self-concept. We have an epiphany that moves from implicit feeling to claimed identity: "I can do this! I am a musical person!" It is the Social Actor in transition to Motivated Agent.

Embodiment as Musical Disposition

In Chapter 1, I introduced the idea that children become the music—the merging of the dancer and the dance—as a way to deepen the experience. This was described by many participants as well.

My friend Ben and I would request that my mother put on a recording of Perlman playing Bazzini's "Dance of the Goblins." We would leap all over the living room—I recall thinking that the music could make me dance across the ceiling. The frenetic energy of the piece and of the performance filled me. It compelled me to move, to run around, to express that music. Even though my parents weren't musical, there was ample music in the home. My parents had an extensive record collection which was an integral part of play for me and my friends. (Nathan, 2009)

Music theorist Thomas Clifton (1983) used the term "possession" to describe this feeling of musical experience, and Nathan's story is a clear example. Possessed by the music, he is "filled" with the performance and it (implicitly) compels him to move. There is a sense of getting lost in music—responding to the analogous relationship between sound and body. When an undefinable implicit feeling is made sonically or physically explicit, the resulting clarity often evokes an elated response. This emotional power of the experience becomes associated with the action and our memory is "tagged" with value.

We not only embody the music; we also embody the musician. This "emulation" is more characteristic of middle childhood, when we are not only Social Actors but are more aware of intensions—we are Motivated Agents of our own identities. Descriptions of "trying on" various musical personas were very common in these autobiographies.

> *My friends would come to my house and we would spend hours playing record after record in the comfort of my bedroom, dancing until we were tired and singing until we were hoarse. You could not tell us that we were not recording stars singing on stage. Here is the reason why. The other significant experience for me was seeing the live shows at the Apollo Theater. I lived within walking distance of the venue and my friends and I would hang out there on the Saturday afternoon and see all of the music legends: Smokey Robinson, (Little) Stevie Wonder, and Marvin Gaye, Pearl Bailey, Nancy Wilson, just to name a few. These were some of the happiest days of my life. (Linda "Lebab," 2016)*

Through recordings, we can become the performer on stage, where the deep knowledge of sound is cultivated through repeated enactments of a single imagined performance. When we engage due to our own volition, we assume agency and claim our identity as musicians.

> *In middle school, I decided that I wanted to do more than just sing along to my favorite artists. One day when listening to a Dave Matthews song, I had an epiphany:* **Wait a second, what if I, Johnny, were one of these musical artists that I love so much?** *The next day, my father took me to Sam Ash to purchase my first instrument, a $150 Fender squire electric guitar. In the basement of my house, I had my personal "rock lair" adorned, including a tiny Marshall amp and microphone stand. I set everything up in front of a large mirror, and in these nascent days of my musicianship, I attempted to master that "rock star" persona as I struggled to strum along to songs on the stereo. I sounded terrible, often not even knowing when the guitar or my voice was out of tune, but it didn't matter, because when I felt the weight of that guitar hang on my shoulders and I pressed my lips to the microphone, I felt like an integral component of the music; far closer to the melody and rhythm than when my parents danced to Paul Simon. I simply felt like I was in the groove, and I didn't want to leave. (Johnny, 2015)*

Dispositions in music are recalled in childhood activities such as exploring musical objects, as in Jessica's picking up the cello, and engaging in pretend play, as in Labab's singing on stage and Johnny's guitar playing. Each of these activities invites focus and attention to the moment. What do those musical dispositions look like in later years? We can see a path vis-à-vis our earliest experiences when we submit to the intensity of being moved by, or as Frith (1996) wrote, getting lost in music. This is followed by emulation of others making music and seeing oneself as a musician, acting as someone is explicitly a "musician." Once our musical identities have been culturally endorsed, we return to the implicit connections to music in the moment, now imbued with explicit knowledge that we can name and address. These are both examples of "fitting in." In the next section, we will examine the experiences of "standing out" and how dispositional traits set us apart and inform our musical selves.

Dispositional Personality Traits and Motivating Conditions

McAdams (2015) identifies three layers of personality that develop over the human lifespan introduced earlier in the chapter. The first to appear, the Social Actor, is present in infancy. The social actor is driven by seeking answers to "How do I act?" and "What do I feel?" and is absorbed in the present; most of the examples provided in the discussion on embodiment are enacted at this level. The second level, Motivated Agent, is infused with intention and an awareness of consequences, and therefore is informed by the present and future. Asking "What do I want?" and "What do I value?," this level usually appears first in middle childhood. The perspective of Autobiographical Author, the third level, is associated with emerging adulthood as we strive to seek answers to monumental questions including "Who am I?," "Who have I been?," and "Who am I becoming?"

To better understand these levels and the ways in which they combine and interact in shaping our musical identities, I begin by reviewing the Big 5 dispositional traits named by McAdams (taken from Goldberg, 1981): Conscientiousness, Extraversion, Openness to New Ideas, Neuroticism, and Agreeableness. The first four were clearly present in the autobiographies included in this study and are used to explore the possible relationships between music dispositions and individual traits. Of the one remaining, Agreeableness, with its positive descriptors of Good-natured, Soft-hearted, Courteous, Forgiving, Sympathetic, and Agreeable, was not a salient theme in these autobiographical accounts of musicians. This trait was valued in teachers but was absent in reflections on the participants' own identity and musical self.

Conscientiousness and Artistry

For the student autobiographers, making music is a motivating condition. The descriptive markers for conscientiousness—well-organized, self-disciplined, and persevering—are usually equated with academic success, but what about musical success? Practicing was clearly an act of conscientiousness in which they linked effort to results, as this student describes:

One of the most memorable songs the jazz band played was the Charles Mingus composition "Haitian Fight Song." I was always struck by the angry nature of the music, but how it was so beautiful at the same time. Another reason I liked playing it was that there was a transcribed Mingus bass solo that I had to learn. Another composition we played was a Duke Ellington song called "Happy Go Lucky Local." This song will always have a special place in my heart because for four months, I only practiced the impossible fast triplet line in the bass solo. This made me realize that if I really practice hard, I can do anything on the instrument. (Jeff, 2013)

In this case, conscientiousness is rewarded with self-efficacy—Jeff can hear and feel his success. The concept of emergent motivation (Csikszentmihalyi & Rathunde, 1993) provides a context for this dispositional trait, for it is when we can see consequential change as a result of our efforts that we are compelled to continue—to be conscientious in our work.

Jeff referred to both the beauty of the piece as well as the technical skill he developed. But how does this trait interact with artistry, musicality, or creativity? The epiphany of one student provides an example of how her conscientiousness was preventing her from meeting her aesthetic goal:

I have been playing the piano for eighteen years. During those years I have had seven piano teachers. I still remember one of my music teachers who really influenced me. . . . One day, I went to the teacher's house to take my piano lesson. At that time, I was playing a piece that mixed angry and anxious feelings. I played it very carefully. I followed the expression markings; I played every note correctly. I felt good and confident. After I played the piece, my teacher told me to continue playing it. Then she left the piano studio. I played and waited. I did not hear any sound from the door. I thought she had already forgotten me. I felt angry, but I could not stop my playing. If I stopped, she might get angry with me. After a period of time, I was not in the mood for following the expression markings carefully, so I used my feelings to play the piece. After she came back, she wanted me to explain the difference between the first time and the last time. Suddenly, I realized that I needed to add my own feelings into a piece. (Hsiao Chin, 1998)

Dispositional traits are complex phenomena. They work in combination with each other and are observable in repeated actions and reactions across contexts. The following discussion of Extraversion shows its very recognizable presence in musical performance.

Extraversion and Performance

Whether music performers are more extraverted or introverted has been a subject of interest for the last forty years. In his study of orchestra musicians, Kemp (1996) described the performers as being prone to introversion, reflective of the interpretive nature and immersive experience associated with playing an instrument. However, a more recent study which looked at Myers-Briggs personality traits across music majors found that the group of musicians were significantly overrepresented in the Extraversion model (Lesiuk, 2019).

According to McAdams, people high in Extraversion are sociable, fun-loving, and spontaneous, one might even say entertaining. For musicians, these descriptors are most evident in approaches to performance, such as this memory from a student who is now a professional opera singer:

One particular year, while I was in first grade, the theme was songs of the 50s—a collection I knew very well given my mother's constant ear for CBS 101.9. In the auditorium one day during a school-wide assembly, the music teacher—Ms. Romano—played all the songs that were to be performed for that year. When she played "16 Candles" by the Crests, I started singing along, and being

> *in the first row, it caught Ms. Romano's attention. She quickly brought her microphone over to me and had me sing into the mic for the whole assembly to hear. The solo was mine, and I was cast to perform it for the Music Festival. The day of the show I can recall wearing blue jeans and a black leather jacket, with my regular first grade teacher . . . using hair gel to slick my hair back and part it. I remember a full auditorium of students, staff and parents, and I also remember having a real darn good time singing to them!* (Constandino, 2012)

Here, the social actor is engaging in imaginary play, his slick-backed hair and leather jacket serving to make the experience authentic. His performance is imbued with optimism that comes from his extraversion. He enjoyed his role as a soloist and embodied the character—a singer with the Crests. A similar disposition for performing is also seen in the excerpt below:

> *In fifth grade, my three best friends and I sang and danced to "Stop in the Name of Love" by the Supremes. A friend and I also emceed the show. My parents like to talk about how shocking it was to see me emcee the show with such confidence and ease. I was an extremely shy and reserved kid most of the time. I remember walking to school with my mom the morning after the performance. She asked me, "What is it like performing like that? Don't you get nervous?" I responded, "No." As I was saying this, I remember feeling very proud. In retrospect, I think this was the moment that I began identifying as a performer.* (Elise, 2015)

Four years younger than Elise in his story, Constandino is the Social Actor, fully enjoying the moment and answering the question "How do I feel?": *"I also remember having a real darn good time singing to them!"* Elise's ability to respond to her mother's question shows the intentional Motivated Agent—she addresses the question of "What do I want?" by later stating *"because when I'm on stage, I can be anyone I want to be!"* Her role as agent is joined by her social actor role, as she also draws attention to her feelings, demonstrating the layers of personality that continue contributing to our identities.

Performing music provides a unique opportunity to engage in extraverted behavior that controls for neuroticism, the temporal, spatial, and expressive qualities of music providing means by which we can temporarily lose the insecurities and worry often associated with being the center of attention. We become immersed in the moment—for children this looks like running and leaping to Bazzini's "Dance of the Goblins." For adults, it may be the rewards of creating—of seeing ideas manifest through artistic practice. They too are immersed—sustaining the impetus to adapt their behavior and thinking to new cues revealed through the openness to possibility.

Openness to Experience

McAdams (2015) lists the following descriptors for the trait of Openness to Experience: Original, Imaginative, Creative, Broad Interests, Complex, and Curious.

Three of these, imagination, creativity, and curiosity, are expressed in memories of childhood music making, with specific and observable associated behaviors that we also recognize in adult musical activity.

To relate this trait to the music experiences described in the data, I offer a longer excerpt from a musician educator who was willing and open to engage in the unknown. As an immigrant to the United States, Tanya was familiar with the idea of change and was willing to try new instrumental experiences.

> *When I moved to America in fourth grade, there was a demonstration of musical instruments at my school. I was so mesmerized because I have never seen instruments before. What beautiful sounds! That day, I went home and asked my mom if I could take lessons at school, and she suggested I play the violin. I loved the violin. The shiny body, the way the chin rest vibrates when I pluck the strings, the dry smell of rosin. From what I could tell at the time, I advanced quickly, but I was no match for students who have been taking private lessons since they were three years old. . . .*
>
> *In sixth grade orchestra one day, Mrs. Ciminnisi asked if anyone would be willing to switch to the bass because we didn't have a bass player. Being curious [about] what a bass even was, I shyly raised my hand, and she said to talk to her after class. Later that week, she put a bass in my hands, and my whole new life began. (Tanya, 2015)*

Due to her openness to new experiences, Tanya was willing to try the bass and eventually was accepted into a major US conservatory as a bass major. In her high school years, she took a chance with another instrument.

> *"Do you know how to play bass guitar?" Mr. Flowers asked. No, I replied. "Good, you'll be performing the Hairspray Medley on it in a few months," he*

> said. I was scared. He expected me to learn a new instrument by practicing a professional Broadway piece. It was like a beginner trying to learn how to play football by playing in the National Football League; it was impossible. I was no longer the star of the field-this was not my territory. . . .
>
> It was late at night in the chorus room. After running through the Hairspray Medley numerous times [over] the past months [and] the past hours, we were exhausted. But as the last note rang from the amp and the piano, we knew we had crossed the finish line. The last note filled my lungs with ecstasy and pride. [Mr. Flowers] smiled and asked, "Impossible? It's improbable, but you did it." The last note still rang, and it encircled my soul. Even though I was tired after toiling for hours, there is nowhere else I would [have] rather been. I've always wanted to go to the exciting country of Japan, or the land of kangaroos in Australia, but forever and always, I will never trade any other moment anywhere else for the moment I fell in love with music.

Here the traits of Conscientiousness and Openness join to create this moment of satisfaction and joy when her musical identity was assured. She continues:

> With my limits surpassed, I performed in the Spring Concert. I plucked my bass guitar and looked at Mr. Flowers bounce his hands up and down on the ivory keys of the piano to the Hairspray Medley. At that moment, I realized that the notes created by our essence had transformed into chords that carried us and the audience into a utopia of music. Within a millisecond of a change in the chord, I had discovered peace and perfection within the music, myself, and the entire world.

Tanya's openness to experience set her first on the path to playing a new instrument, which, in turn, led to contexts that affirmed her connections to the "entire world."

Neuroticism and the Vulnerability of Emotional Expression

The descriptors of Neuroticism, or what has also been called "negative emotionality," include worrying, nervous, high-strung, insecure, and vulnerable (McAdams, 2015). The emotional nature of musical performance often provoked the use of intense language to describe these musicians' experiences. In Tanya's story she shares, "*I was scared*," suggesting worrying and insecurity. Yet, this memory is countered by the following statements that from her come later in her story:

"The last note filled my lungs with ecstasy and pride."
"... chords that carried us and the audience into a utopia of music"
"I have discovered peace and perfection within the music, myself, and the entire world."

Such intense language conveys a depth of feeling that mediated the one condition of neuroticism and demonstrates that musical experiences can be sites for resilience and transcendence (see Chapter 5).

In an interview study of professional musicians on their experiences of becoming a musician, Wiggins (2011) found agency and vulnerability to be key themes. She found vulnerability to be experienced both positive and negative consequences. The positive effects were interpreted in the discussion on "Openness to Experience"—Tanya did make herself vulnerable in taking on the unknown, and it led to rewarding outcomes. Wiggins attributes the negative effects of vulnerability to the nature of music as a sonic and therefore public activity susceptible to judgment. Indeed, in this group of music students, there existed a context in which the worrying, insecurities, and vulnerabilities that define this disposition appeared. These involved a self-image based on comparisons with others; such feelings were often a result of teaching practices based on competition.

The prospect of attending a music junior high school was the musical foundation it gave me and the psychological strength I gained from the experiences in performing. The negative side was comprehending music as a competition. The school was always involved in some kind of competition, and it was our responsibility to do well in these events. One day you would be working as a team with your classmates, and other days you are competing against them. This created tension, stress, and lack of confidence among students. (Mizuki, 2005)

Below, read how one student recalls her youthful experiences. Her struggles were with competition, and her anxiety about performance was more about revealing her private inner feelings than with making technical errors. Note the use of words suggesting negative emotions: competitive, worry, anxiety, tension, betrayal, frustration, and confrontation.

> *My indulgence into moody and sorrowful music was enhanced after I entered music school (middle school). My school was extremely competitive, and I got easily hurt by my friends (even best friends) lying about how many hours they practiced. As an adolescent, I felt betrayed by people I trusted. At that time, I always listened to music which sounded very tragic such as Albinoni's "Adagio in g minor," Verdi's opera overture from "La Forza del Destino," and Brahms's "Symphony no. 3." Those pieces seemed to express my frustration, feelings of being betrayed by reality as well as my anxiety in becoming a great violinist. While I was listening to those pieces, I created a confrontation in my destiny. It was a confrontation between my desire to become a musician and failing to become [one]. . . .*
>
> *After I entered university, I had a lot of chances to perform in public. I loved being on the stage because it felt so real and alive. Tension is not abstract like studying. As I got used to tension on the stage, I began to enjoy the different feeling of time and space on the stage. . . . Music is a way to travel to another dimension. Playing music (especially very sorrowful music) has been a secret gate to my own world. Opening this gate has helped me see the relationships between who I am, who I think I am, and who others think I am. Now I know that all of these are parts of me. Music explains the way I live and how I communicate with myself and others. Sometimes I worry that the audience will sense my secret melancholy. I have become accustomed to my outward image of brightness and innocence. Part of me wants to protect this from being disclosed. At the same time, I want to convey a cleansing of genuine emotion to others. (Heejung, 1999)*

Heejung's memory also reflects the creativity and complexity of thought found in Openness to Experience; McAdams (2015) cites research that the development of this trait is likely tied up with factors that "influence one's sensitivity to internal and external sensory stimulation" (p. 107). Her sensitivity to the time and space of musical performance may provide buttressing of the negative emotions mentioned above.

There were a few students whose expressed experiences with competition were motivating and had positive consequences.

The first pleasant musical experience I ever had was when I was in junior high school. I used to compete with my best friend. I always practiced hard on the piano so that I could beat my friend. The competition motivated me to practice the piano and to improve my piano skills. After my friend moved away, I stopped playing the piano because I did not have any [reason]. . . . Then I came to the United States. I started to practice the piano again when I met a new friend in tenth grade. We both enrolled in the piano school where I experienced the second pleasant moment playing piano. She and I always competed just like when I was in junior high school. (Gemma, 1999)

Dispositional traits help define how we experience music and "how we are" with certain musical practices. In the next sections, I examine "How do we belong to music?" through excerpts about the choice of instrument, the presence of musical models, and the relationships with peers.

Instrument Choice and Identity

"A New Friend"

I was so excited to learn a "real" instrument for the first time, and had my eyes set on the trumpet. I remember taking it home for the first time and opening up the case. Though it was used and in mediocre condition, I can remember treating it as if it were made of solid gold. This memory . . . now feels much like those memories I have of meeting friends for the first time. Music had always made me feel safe, but for the first time I also felt exhilaration and a sense of real potential. (Berkley, 2012)

There are many reasons individuals end up playing a specific instrument. It is determined by socially prevalent stereotyping dealing with gender (Abeles & Porter, 1978; Abeles, 2009) as well as a player's physical size and home culture. There are circumstances such as accessibility (the family owns a clarinet) or convenience (a drum teacher lives next door). In whatever way the choice was made, music education students wrote much about their connections to specific musical instruments. Many, like Berkley, spoke with a reverence for the object.

> *My first vivid musical memories are from the third grade. I remember walking down the hall to music class on the day we were given our recorders. It was a good day. I was overjoyed to have an instrument of my own. I remember taking it apart and putting it back together, cleaning it and putting it away. I loved that it had its own case and cleaning supplies. That night, I brought it to a restaurant when my parents took us out to dinner. I couldn't bear to part with it. . . .*
>
> *The day I got my flute in fourth grade was even more exciting. . . . It had so many buttons and parts; the possibilities seemed endless. That year, the high school band played an assembly for us and talked about the different instruments. The performance was inspiring. I let my imagination go wild as I listened. At the end of the concert, the director asked all the fourth grade band students to stand up when their instrument was called. I was overcome with pride as I stood with the flute group. It was the first time I had identified myself as an instrumentalist. (Zoe, 2013)*

Others like Cynthia, below, wrote about taking a chance with something she knew little about, and magically, it was a perfect match:

> *As I moved up in elementary school, and into the fourth and fifth grade building, I was able to start learning an instrument. Because of a slight overbite, I was told to choose a brass instrument or the drums, and chose the trombone because it sounded interesting, and I didn't quite know what it was . . . when I chose the trombone, I was very glad it was not a flute (which my sister also played), and the fact that she couldn't get a note to sound good on MY instrument was very fulfilling.*
>
> *My trombone and I have been through a lot since then, and I am very glad I chose it. . . . I joined the fifth grade band while I was still in the fourth grade because I had "talent," and was very proud of that. From that point on I was in love. I was always considered very important in the band because there were only three trombones, as opposed to a million and one flutes, and the fact that the boys teased me as I carried my instrument on the bus and into school did not really bother me. Besides, I could always swing the hard case and "accidentally" hit them in the back. (Cynthia, 2001)*

For some there was an attraction that was a mystery—a possible series of random experiences that served to expose them to the instrument and somehow captured their imagination.

I have always wanted to be a violinist. I cannot remember an age where the instrument did not fascinate me. I can, however, remember that at a very young age, I would waltz across my home with two curtain rods using one as a very thin fiddle and the other as its bow.

My parents and I often reflect on that moment wondering where I had gotten such a notion to play. No one in my family was a violinist so where had I seen or heard the instrument? . . . I know my mother encouraged musical play very early on. I loved to dance around with a microphone and make up silly songs and you could not keep me away from the piano! One of the songs my mom and I composed on the way to school one day actually won a contest and was played on the local radio station. Yet, there were no violins with which to experiment. I had certainly seen and heard the instrument somewhere. I clearly remember seeing Big Bird talking to a Suzuki violin student on Sesame Street. I also recall seeing Itzak Perlman introduce the violin to one of my favorite 80s characters, Punky Brewster. Even with these colorful memories, I think the most impressionable moments of the violin came from a more active experience. The excitement of my mother's concerts must have encouraged my interests in music, and more specifically, the violin and orchestral studies. (Amy, 2004)

This mystery of exposure takes us back to the idea of implicit learning. These early experiences can have consequences of which we are unaware, until some cue in the present environment awakens the memory. Several of the autobiographers commented on how spending the time examining their past led to more questions about how their current lives might be different had certain decisions not been made.

Access: What If . . . ?

A few students found themselves wondering about how their musical lives might have been different had they made or been given other choices or opportunities.

At the beginning of sixth grade, we were tested in four areas: singing, band, acting, and art. Based on the results, the school then placed us on a three-year track that included participation in one of these subjects for four periods a week. I wanted band more than anything, despite the fact that I had primarily sung my entire life. Something about it called to me. Perhaps it was the fact that I had never done anything like it, or maybe it was because I had watched my brothers play instruments. This I cannot remember for sure, but I do recall how devastated I felt when they put me in chorus due to my lack of instrumental experience. In fact, the first and only instrument I truly remember playing was a very small piano that only had one octave. It probably didn't sound very good, but my mother taught me to play chopsticks on it. I was extremely proud when I finally learned the song and every so often, I revisit the tune to make sure I still remember it, despite its simplicity. I have thought back to that rejection from band often. Where would I be if I had started playing trumpet, or sax, or percussion? Would I be better off, or would music not have impacted me the same way it did later? (Jenna, 2012)

Students also considered the "goodness of fit" in their experiences with particular instruments:

At about the same time, I quit playing the piano and switched to violin. I was fed up with the same melodies and materials all of my friends played in the piano institute. Everybody played pieces from Viel or Czerny which I could not stand listening to anymore. The instrument itself (piano) was just not enough to express my overwhelming emotion and too mechanical to get close to. I was very excited about learning how to play the violin because violin was small enough to manage by myself and I could transpose any song I knew without looking at a complicated score. Also, the most important aspect was that the violin could produce more melancholy and expressive sounds with vibrato which piano does not have at all! (Heejung, 1999)

This memory and the present-day questions asked by the student reflect the doubt and curiosity we each have about what is, what was, and what will be. These excerpts also serve to remind us of the varied backgrounds and dispositions each student carries with them.

Finding Musical Kin

"We Looked Somewhat Similar"

I remember the first time I read an academic book that used feminine pronouns. It was David Hargreaves's book on musical development; the year was 1992. I was surprised at how strongly it affected me—I had this overwhelming new feeling as though someone was actually referring to me. That spirit of kinship has much to do with our identities, and we seek affinity with others that are like us.

In the United States, classical music (or Western art music) has been historically considered the music of the white upper class, and until recently, there were few Black performers in classical orchestras or on opera stages (DeLorenzo, 2012). One of the first to break through these barriers and be recognized in the classical field was the great Marian Anderson, who writes about the realization of possibility in her autobiography, *My Lord, What a Morning*:

> When I was about eight years old Father got us a piano. . . . I did not have lessons; there was not enough money for a teacher. However, we did acquire from somewhere a card, marked with the notes, that one could set up directly back of the keys. With the help of this, we learned some simple melodies. But it did not occur to me, that I could learn to play the piano properly. I was walking down the street one day, carrying a basket of laundry that I was delivering for my mother, when I heard the sound of the piano. I sat down my basket, went up the steps and looked into the window. I knew it was wrong to peep, but I could not resist the temptation. I saw a woman seated at a piano, playing ever so beautifully. Her skin was dark like mine. I realized that if she could, I could. (1956, pp. 12–13)

"If she could, I could." The importance of relatable models cannot be overstated. Such kinship was expressed by several music educators in this study.

> *By the age of six, I was more aware that I did not look like the other members in my family. (By the time I turned six years old, my mother had given birth to my two younger sisters). I lived in a predominantly white town with very little diversity, and my classmates began asking questions about my "real family" and my "real parents." I remember feeling frustrated because I did not know how to respond to their questions. One night, I was watching a special on PBS with my family and violin soloist Sarah Chang performed a violin concerto. I felt extremely connected to the music and her playing, but also at the fact that she was Asian and we looked somewhat similar. After her performance, I told my parents that I wanted to play the violin. I felt a connection with Sarah Chang that I had not felt before and was completely set on learning how*

to play the violin. My parents were apprehensive about me learning a new instrument since I was already taking piano lessons, but after several months of asking them repeatedly, they finally decided to let me try. (Liz, 2000)

The power of seeing ourselves represented as musicians gives us power to claim the identities we imagine.

In addition to teaching us Broadway musicals, Mrs. McLoud would take a group of us to Lincoln Center every year to see The Nutcracker performed by the New York City Ballet. Although the dance numbers were beautifully executed, it was Pyotr Ilyich Tchaikovsky's musical score that I fell in love with. The sounds coming from the orchestra pit: horns, flutes, clarinets, violins, harps, and large drums were enchanting. I had never heard these instruments played together to produce this sound called classical music. I was fascinated. It was not until I was in fifth grade that those same instruments finally made their way into our school. Along with the instruments came two music teachers, Misters Alvin and Ed Pazant. They were brothers and they were African American. It was the first time we saw African American men in our school in the role of a teacher and that excited us. Ed Pazant played the alto saxophone and taught the woodwind instruments, and Alvin Pazant played the trumpet and taught the brass instruments. I was assigned the French horn by Alvin Pazant and I never understood (or questioned) why. The horn weighed almost as much as I did, as I was a very skinny little girl. Still, I was very excited to be given the opportunity to learn a "grown-up" instrument. Ed and Alvin Pazant also took a special interest in the students. They volunteered to give lessons in their free time to students who were struggling with their instrument. By the time I graduated from elementary school I had a few school performances under my belt, I was singing better, I was learning an instrument, I had a love of two new music genres, and I had decided that I wanted music to be a constant in my life. For many of us these music experiences were life-changing, even life-saving. Music has the power to do that. For some of us who might otherwise have been pulled into the negative activities in the Harlem streets when we were older, music pulled us in a different direction and kept us focused. Thank you, Mrs. McLoud and Misters Ed and Alvin Pazant. (Lebab, 2016)

The experiences of having two new music genres and being taught by people who looked like her led Lebab to claim her musical identity, "*to have music as a constant in my life.*"

Performing Kinship: Playing Together

Collective musical experiences are the driving motivation for a sustained engagement with performing and an identity in music. This happens throughout the lifespan, beginning with infant-parent vocalized dialogues to membership in the New Horizon band programs for adult seniors.

In this first excerpt, the student recalls how playing in the orchestra provided experiences that highlighted what it meant to be a musician. She was something of a prodigy, starting the violin at age three, and by age five she had won a competition and was touring with her Suzuki group internationally.

When I was nine years old, I was enrolled in the Julliard Pre-college Division. Reflecting back to these years, I do not [have] many good memories. I remember being placed in a theory class that was much too advanced for me. I was extremely intimidated and completely lost. Even violin lessons were not pleasant experiences. My teacher was very strict. She would get impatient when I didn't understand. As a result, I would get stomachaches whenever I was nervous or fearful. I wasn't very motivated to practice, because playing the violin wasn't fun. Although these experiences were difficult, I still loved music. In this program I was given the opportunity to play in an orchestra. This was a totally new experience for me, and I believe that this helped shape the way I think about music. I remember the very first orchestra piece I played was "Eine kleine Nachtmusik." I was in awe about how beautiful the harmony [was] and [about] the sound of all the instruments meshed together. This was something that I looked forward to every Saturday. I think for the first time I heard music not just with my ears, but with my heart. (Susan, 1999)

Compare Susan's words to the recollections of an experience during the college years from this student:

When I was attending NEC, my friend Caroline invited me to join a chamber orchestra for a concert tour in Germany. We practiced, ate delicious foods, and traveled all throughout the country giving concerts. One of the pieces we performed was Verklärte Nacht by Schoenberg on Roseninsel (Rose Island). Peter Joseph Lenné designed the garden for King Maximilian II of Bavaria and it was a beautiful island filled with a massive garden filled with varieties of roses. **I still remember the feeling I felt as we played through this complex piece of music. We captured the essence of the poem, creating splashes of** *color and texture through our performance together.* When we finished the last note, there was a roar of applause and the audience gave us a standing ovation. We were immersed in the energy in the concert hall and knew that we had created a special musical experience together. It is moments like these that make me remember and appreciate why I love music, the collaborative effort of preparing and making music, and sharing our passions with others. (Kokoe, 2016)

Such descriptions of transcendence were common in stories of ensemble playing. So were stories of mutuality. These last two excerpts demonstrate what can happen when we see ourselves in another:

The youth orchestra I was in was going to Israel. . . . From the first day of the tour, I started to make new friends, and through the concerts, I was deeply moved by my fellow musicians. We played "New World Symphony" by Dvořák, amongst other pieces. As the title indicated, it opened my eyes to a whole new world of music. We played nine concerts there, and the students participated in all rehearsals and all concerts enthusiastically. I was impressed by how serious they were, and how much they loved music. . . . By the ninth concert, everyone in the orchestra memorized the whole piece, and we all played the concert by memory. It was the most remarkable moment. I realized I was very lucky to be there with them. Now, I had a burning desire to learn and study more about music and the cello. (Sooyoung Lee, 1999)

This trip with the youth orchestra provided Sooyoung opportunity for musical kinship—she found people who were passionate about making music, which ignited "a burning desire to learn and study more about music and the cello." In the example below, the autobiographer finds mutuality with others in the shared need for challenge:

I attended Campus Middle [School] for one year from age thirteen to fourteen. While there I participated in the school's concert band and jazz band. The level of the music program there was considerably lower than what I was accustomed to in Minnesota and motivated me to seek out alterative outlets for my musical needs outside of school. I joined the Colorado Youth Symphony, and the Colorado Honor Band, and after finishing my year . . . I went to Telluride Jazz Camp during the summer. While there, I, for the first time, met other kids who were like me—felt underchallenged by their school music programs. I met

Pat Blodgett there, who became my private trombone teacher for the next four years and formed alliances there with other kids from schools all around the Denver area. (Gary, 1998)

Relationships with others are key drivers in the development of musical identity. The role of human interactions starts in infancy with the communicative musicality of parent-child vocalizations and continues into childhood with imaginative musical play with friends. By early adolescence we affiliate with others with whom we share musical preferences and dispositional traits. In the final section of this chapter, I summarize the ways we come to identify ourselves as musicians and how, as Autobiographical Authors, we make explicit the implicit knowledge of our past as it pertains to our present and future.

A Sense of Musical Self

Positionality in the Formation of Musical Identity

In musical activity, as well as in other performing arts such as dance and theater, we can engage in both individual and collective experiences and maintain an authentic representation of the art form. This characteristic of generous inclusion—a welcoming of the soloist and the ensemble player— was present in the autobiographies and provided examples of multiple entry points for meaningful participation.

Heejung described her performing as a "way to travel to another dimension" and to take her audience along—her entry point to musicianship was through individual expression. She was concerned, however that by conveying emotion, she was vulnerable to exposure of feelings she didn't want to share. This identity of emotional conduit was also present in her decision to change from the piano to the violin, with which she could share a greater range of intensity and sentiment.

Compare this to the collective experiences shared by Susan, Kokoe, and Sooyoung, for whom the opportunity to share their passion for performing with other musicians in orchestral settings was at the forefront of their memories. For these musicians, the social value of music making may be defined differently; however, fitting in and standing out are not experienced as binaries. They are under constant negotiation: considering individual and collective positionalities is something all musicians do, and the recollections of those experiences when we were called to modify our musical selves to achieve shared musical outcomes are very strong. Identities are malleable and change because of interactions with others (Randall, 2015).

Other entry points involved the attraction to a specific type of musical instrument, and the realization that it was a good fit for the musician. This was voiced by many of the autobiographers. Upon opening his trumpet case for the first time, Berkley felt "exhilaration" and a "sense of real potential." Very early on, students became identified with their instruments, and students like Cynthia, who wrote, "I was always considered very important in the band because there were only three trombones, as opposed to a million and one flutes . . .," embraced this identity. Yet, there were also stories of struggle from musicians like Jenna, who was denied an opportunity to explore her identity as an instrumentalist. I do want to point out that the participant demographics of this sample to some extent controlled for inequities in musical prospects—this group of music educators was enrolled in a graduate program at an Ivy League institution that required some type of performance background and an undergraduate degree in music. (See Chapter 5 for student stories of disruption, change, and renewal of musical trajectories.)

Musical identities were strongly connected to feelings of belonging with musical groups. Singing in choirs was the most common ensemble experience mentioned in the autobiographies, which harkens back to earlier interactions with family, where singing was a primary communicative tool for social bonding. These were followed by descriptions of belonging to instrumental groups—most references were to orchestra or band settings. However, a surprising number mentioned jazz band as a setting that offered a connection to playing or singing that was musically genuine. The foundational practices of jazz performance include the constant negotiation of individual and collective contributions of solo and tutti, and its characteristic improvisation, which mimics the nature of music making as it moves between the implicitly retrieved creation in the moment and the explicitly rendered score.

Musical Identity and Dispositional Traits

Earlier in this chapter we reviewed four of McAdams's (2015) five dispositional traits and how they may help interpret memories of how we become musicians. Our subject, musical identity, is situated in memories of active music making over the lifespan, and although we have some personal traits that are stable, our dispositions can change bidirectionally: past experiences affect present actions, and as Autobiographical Authors, our present contexts influence our recollections of memories. Music's role in human development, from both evolutionary (Wallin, Merker, & Brown, 2001) and ontogenetic viewpoints (Trehub, 2001), is adaptive and ever-changing.

To honor the complexity of the musical self, the most useful application of these traits is looking at them in combination to see how they interact to facilitate (and interfere with) musical production and response. The trait McAdams calls Open to New Experiences (O) was the most influential, especially in regard to keeping in check the negative emotionality of Neuroticism (N) present in so many music performance settings. Tanya, who had a very high level of O, was able to feign off the feeling of being scared because of her ability to imagine what could be. A high level of Conscientiousness (C) helped her be able to take advantage of the resources offered in her "new experience." Heejung, on the other hand, started with a high N and was able to mediate its effects through her use of strategies defining the O trait. It may be that openness to new experiences, like the quality Csikszentmihalyi and Getzels (1988) called "discovery orientation," is a favored dispositional trait in artists.

There were elements of musical identity that were not directly addressed in McAdams's Big Five. Relatable to Openness to New Experiences, the attraction to the challenges that music engagement provides, and the recognition that musicians have the ability to meet those challenges, is mentioned in a majority of the stories told. When challenges are aligned with perceived skills, there is a feeling of growth and discovery that perpetuates successful movement toward a clear goal. Jeff discussed such a feeling when he recognized that if he practiced hard, he could do anything. Tanya spoke of meeting the challenges and the ultimate rewards of playing new music. Cynthia conveyed her pride in being elevated to fifth grade band while still in fourth grade. And Gary found refuge in a group of musicians who had the same hunger for being highly challenged as he did. Each of these students identified as musicians because they could read the evidence in their actions.

5

Musical Pathways

Disruption and Renewal in Musical Lives

My college years were some of the hardest times that I have encountered so far. I felt as though I did not know my own identity and I struggled with the meaning of my music. It was during this dry period when I experienced the power of music for the first time. I was beginning to understand the power of music; the way it spoke from the heart of the performer to the heart of the listener. In 1994 I had the awesome privilege of working with a piano trio, and this became the turning point in my life. I renewed my passion and love for music making. (Elisa, 1999)

Elisa started playing piano at age three. She was concertizing and entering international competitions by middle childhood and attended the Juilliard pre-college program at age fifteen, eventually earning her bachelor's and master's degrees from the same institution. With this illustrious past, it seems that her path was well-defined; however, at one point, she was called to question her present identity and to reconcile the meaning of her past experiences with her existing circumstances. This disruption was a seemingly necessary process. After so much time focusing on a solo career and being surrounded by peers who had made similar choices at an institution where individual performers were celebrated, it was collective music making that brought her renewal. As was seen in the previous chapter, it was common for memories of middle childhood to include such "Ah ha!" moments when finding kin, that is, people with shared musical passion and values.

Road Trips

Previously, we looked at music and the interactions between dispositions and musical contexts and how they created musical identity, especially in middle childhood and early adolescence. This chapter examines graduate music education students' memories across the lifespan, from childhood to late adolescence and early adulthood, specifically looking at the paths they forged to get to their present circumstance, and the expected and unexpected changes that led them there. For most, this meant disruptions and renewals in musician professional trajectories that were caused or repaired by a change in teacher, instrument, or institution. For disruptions in personal lives, such as traumatic loss of a loved one or physical trauma and illness, music could serve as a mode of healing, but also as a source of further pain.

In addition to viewing our paths as a series of changes that impacted direction over a period of time, I also draw upon McAdams's (2015) seven common dimensions of narratives (introduced in Chapter 2), which suggest motivational purpose and serve to explain outcomes in autobiographical work. They include Redemption, Agency, Communion, Contamination, Coherence, Complexity, and Meaning Making. In my analysis of the autobiographies of music teachers, I found multiple dimensions operating. The above excerpt from Elise's story, for example, could be interpreted as a "Redemption Narrative," as it focuses on a "demonstrably 'bad' or emotionally negative event or circumstance that leads to a demonstrably 'good' or positive outcome" (p. 265). The initial negative state is "redeemed" or salvaged by the good that follows it. However, there are also elements of Communion in her story, as in the work with her trio.

Using these dimensions along with trajectories of disruption and renewal, I attempt to address music's capability to both reroute and reconnect individuals, and to expose the concomitant vulnerabilities of artistic aspirations. To capture the nature of provoked and evolving change, I present complete narratives[1] from four students' stories.

Disruption and Renewal of Musical Plans

It has been said that change is the only constant in our lives. This can be seen in the trajectories of music educators as they negotiate career paths

---

[1] The autobiographies have been edited to remove short passages that were not considered crucial to the stories. Authors have reviewed and approved these versions.

and personal growth. As adults, memories help us understand/construct the present and project the future. From early childhood to adulthood, there were reported memories and descriptions of the present that were especially influential and valued. The students were, for the most part, feeling good about the trajectories that eventually brought them to graduate school and careers in music education, although each pathway was unique.

Changes in the path were sometimes a result of purposeful choices, while some were a result of decisions made by others. Jenna, whose denied entry into the school band was shared in the previous chapter, had a brother who taught her to play the guitar. She made her own rock band and ended up taking leadership roles in musical productions in high school—hers is an agentic narrative, as she demonstrated by taking control of musical opportunities and blazing her own musical trail.

Another student left high school having been a marching band drum leader and composer-arranger and entered a prestigious Ivy League university to study composition and music theory. Described as an analytic and cerebral program, he felt music had become institutionalized and detached. What he had predicted to be a "flourishing trajectory" turned out differently; however, his determination to recapture the past joy he experienced through music and to remediate the detachment that he was feeling led to his becoming an educator. This narrative is suggestive of McAdams's contamination dimension, where a positively defined event (or experience)—here, music making—turns negative and "erases the effects of the preceding positivity." However, the preceding positivity was resilient to the negative experience, and the story ends up being redemptive.

Occasionally, the early predictions of trajectory are realized. One such example is Patrice, who, as a beginning doctoral student in 2005, wrote her "Musical History," sharing that her main church playing began at age twelve and grew into her directing, composing, performing, and teaching the congregation. She wrote, "During this time, I realized that my religious calling was to be a full-time minister of music, probably at a large Black Baptist church in a metropolitan city." In 2018 she took on such a position at Ebenezer Baptist Church in Atlanta, home church of Martin Luther King Jr.—the first female to ever serve in that post. Yet even Patrice's path included some "off-road" excursions; however, these weren't disruptions, but instead were side trips which enhanced the journey. These included working with Jazz at Lincoln

Center both as a performer and educator, singing with the Broadway Voices choir, and international Gospel tours to Mexico, Brazil, Chile, and Italy.

Next, I present four full autobiographies, each with its own trajectory. There are a multitude of factors that intersect to create the tone and content of these personal stories. These include access to music instruction, dispositional traits, family background, race and ethnicity, gender and sexual orientation, and teaching experience. Recall is dependent upon the zeitgeist in which memories were reported; the chosen narratives were written in 1999, 2010, and 2016, when students were in the beginning stages of either master's or doctoral work in music education and were composed in the context of a class assignment. In choosing these four narratives, my aim was to offer a wide variety of experiences with hopes that readers might find something familiar in the voices of these students. The purpose was not to represent any specific group, but to demonstrate the complexity of the narrative process.

Clara (1999)

Clara's story represents several themes that were common across the spectrum of autobiographies, most notably the influence of parents, teachers, and peers. Below, she begins with her first teacher, when she was six years old, and traces the relationships and their effect on her musical growth:

> *I remember very vividly from the time I started to take piano lessons. This "professor" came to our house and taught me; the first few lessons were fun—then I slowly started to hate playing the piano. She gave me too much homework and I just wanted to go outside and play. Once in a while, when there was a piece I liked, I practiced very hard. Knowing I could play well when I practiced made the professor be even more hard on me. Pretty soon I ended up crying after every lesson. This ordeal ended after about a year.*

This parental intervention was one of several which played a role in her musical life.

> *For about six months I had no piano teacher but played it on my own for fun. I think my parents and I all knew that the problem was the teacher, not the piano. My mother soon got me a new teacher, which worked marvelously,*

and I started to show some real progress. I studied with this teacher for about three years, and she recommended that I major in piano for junior high. Around this time, I also started to take flute lessons. My mother is also responsible for this, she thought it would be fun. I loved flute more than playing the piano—this instrument I, myself, wanted to pursue seriously, but due to being "lightheaded" after long practices, it never worked out. In fourth grade, I started to play the cello. This was also my mother's idea, she once again thought it would be fun! I fell in love with cello right away, the sounds the shape, and just everything about it. I also had an amazing teacher, Mr. Cho, who meant so much to me. I practiced really hard (for that age) and there was a rapid progress. My teacher had big dreams for me, and he was making plans for my future and goals. Of course, my parents weren't too enthusiastic, because they wanted me to just enjoy music and have some other profession for a career. After about two years Mr. Cho died of cancer. During this time, I went through a major depression, not playing the cello for about a year. I was completely lost without him. In junior high I bounced back, practicing again—I really wanted to become a cellist more than ever before. I wanted to pursue my teacher's dream and belief in me by becoming a great cellist.

Here, the shared musical performance dreams of both teacher and student were completely disrupted. Since these dreams were not shared with her parents, Clara had to be her own advocate, conscientiously working to achieve those dreams with a renewed sense of purpose.

As years passed by this goal became more and more difficult. My parents' opposition became stronger, and I went through countless different teachers in one year. Through numerous arguments, I finally convinced my parents to give me a chance in doing what I wanted to do. When I was in eighth grade, I enrolled in the pre-college program at the Juilliard School. Here I met a great teacher who worked hard with me. Soon I entered high school and I started to enter major competitions and play on public concert series. Through many experiences of happiness and disappointments, I think this is when I started to taste the real music world. I went on to Yale University's School of Music, where I worked very hard for maybe the first two years. I had many friends who were much older than me and I started to worry about jobs and future along with them. Until this point all I knew about classical music was the famous soloists. Being with older friends made me face the reality and at the same time I lost big dreams I had for my music career. I probably went through a period of just "wandering," not working very hard and unable to concentrate.

At this juncture in her journey, Clara is experiencing disruption, this time through interactions with peers. Self-doubt, fueled by opinions from people that she trusted, caused her to critically examine her future from a "realistic" perspective that shunned the notion of dreaming of something perhaps not achievable. She was able to renew her commitment to a musical life through the support of a teacher.

Then I went to Boston and was lucky to have met a great teacher. I slowly recovered from my depression and became once again enthusiastic about being a musician. This teacher was great in a way that he was very practical but at the same time inspiring. When I had decided to come to Teachers College, he was very supportive, unlike many of my previous teachers who still feel that being a soloist is the only way. From my experiences, I know the importance of teachers, and how they can alter one's path. (Clara, 1999)

There are many twists and turns in Clara's pathway. Teachers played a significant role in the trajectory she followed, through passion either shared or withheld. It is also clear that Clara is seeking coherence with this subject in her narrative, as she addresses "the importance of teachers" in her final sentence at a point in time when she has newly committed to a teaching career.

Jeremy (2016)

In the following autobiographical story, Jeremy traces the path of his musical life, mindful of the role music making itself—especially singing—plays in the construction of his narrative. Having suffered traumatic losses early on in his journey, his experience highlights the importance of parents, teachers, and peers as sources of both disruption and renewal.

As the youngest of five children, I remember growing up in a household full of sounds. As a result of being culturally [diverse], my family exposed me to all types of music. My mother was African American . . . and my father was from Puerto Rico (European/Afro/Indian). . . . Sundays in our home were known for [my mother] blaring gospel music at the loudest decibel, "cleaning

> house," and getting ready for an epic dinner that took all day to prepare. Looking back, I should consider the relationship between the loudness of our music and God as a form of communication and atonement for our sins. The louder the music, the more God would hear and see that we were a good Christian family! My father's ... choices of music were salsa, boleros, and rock & roll. To this day I remember hearing the sounds of R&B and soul music sounding from the gap from under my bedroom door. Those times typically happened at night when people, alcohol, and perhaps drugs were in company. Whatever was going on, I remember wanting to be a part of the action and the laughter.... The howling and roar from a joke being told, or calamity that ensued from beyond my bedroom door was as exciting as a roller coaster ride that kept me on the edge of my seat....
>
> My musical contribution in our home came by way of singing, banging on our very old and ratty electric organ, or playing my very elegant and colorful Little Tikes™ xylophone piano that only had four keys. Since before kindergarten, I remember being encouraged to sing "church songs," which I learned by rote, to play a magical organ to entertain myself, or play my xylophone piano in a concert exclusive for my siblings. At that time, I thought I was a star, and in many ways I was. I was a star to the family that loved me and cultivated my love for them and for music.

These early descriptions suggest a musical family environment. However, from age five, he and his brother experienced a dramatic disruption and "were sent away to live with an estranged aunt I hardly knew hundreds of miles away from the only home I've ever known." Although his circumstances had changed, Jeremy was able to find positive aspects of this uprooting.

> My Sundays no longer included blaring gospel music from a stereo. I got my gospel fix from the church band that played at every church function. Coincidentally, the reverend and his wife were another uncle and aunt whom I grew to love. I remember my uncle had this electric bass that seemed like the voice of God. He would be at the podium or microphone preaching in one moment and playing the bass in another. And although the music was devout, the sound of the band felt more like old soul then it did Christian. Imagine, singing praises to a higher being and feeling the spirit of the music and sitting to the point where you cannot sit still any longer and the only thing you could do was dance. That was what I experienced every time I attended church, any day of the week.

These early experiences in church with an extended family were foundational for Jeremy—he was transported from the everyday to the ethereal through singing. The soulful musical proficiency he demonstrated early on became a primary resource for him throughout his life.

> *In kindergarten, I was insecure about my speech . . . and hardly participated in class. But that all changed when I was given the opportunity to sing a solo during a Christmas concert the school was putting on for the community. The song was "Jingle Bell Rock." I had never heard this song in my life, yet it was one of the coolest songs I remember ever hearing. I felt so alive on stage singing it and for the first time, I wasn't shy about my voice and the way in which I spoke. Singing was the form of expression that made me feel the most comfortable in a school setting. It was like singing in church, freeing and expressive. Most of all, I was encouraged and supported, just like my aunt had done in church, and just like my mom did back home. I guess that part of home never left me and all had not been destroyed, I still had singing to keep me rooted and secure.*

As an Autobiographical Author, Jeremy recognizes that early on, from his first year in school, his narrative is constructed around music making. Music offered him a chance to be immersed in the present, temporarily relieving the debilitating circumstances he faced.

> *Living in New Jersey again, things were very different. My parents were still in court disputing custody arrangement, so I'd live between my parents' homes. Not only did my grades suffer, but my mental stability. I became depressed and suicidal. . . . I felt I had nothing to live for . . . my parents decided it was best that I lived with my mother full-time. I saw my father on the weekends only. This was a tough time for me.*
>
> *At this point in time, I also started to discover my sexual attraction to boys. I didn't even know what the term "gay" meant, but other kids knew. As a result of my shyness and feminine mannerisms, I was bullied from the fifth grade to the time I was in high school. The depression continued, and so did the suicidal thoughts. I could not escape the torture I experienced in school. The only thing that I truly loved about school were its music classes. The teacher was a much older white man, with a heart of gold. He asked me what instrument I wanted to play and I told him the flute . . . most of the instruments the school owned were broken or needed replacing. With the limited resources, he did the best he could.*

The next year, he was replaced by a teacher who was more choral focused, so instead of band, mostly all students took choir. It was then that I felt something familiar and safe. I flocked to this teacher and his lessons almost instantly. And although I was made fun of for playing a "female" or feminine instrument, no one would make fun of me singing in the choir. I was encouraged and complimented. And again, was given an opportunity to sing a solo at a school performance. Singing had become a vehicle of expression I could depend on when I needed encouragement, it would become the best friend I needed to tell my secrets to and confide in. I could rely on singing to get through some tough times; it was when I was older that I realized how true this statement would be.

I attended Rosa L. Parks School of the Fine and Performing Arts for high school. The school specialized in many art disciplines that ranged from creative writing to drama to music. My major was vocal music. It seemed fitting, being that singing was a safety net of sorts throughout my adolescence. During my four years there, I experienced so many great opportunities, such as singing at Carnegie Hall and West Point Military Base with the New York Pops under the direction of the late Skitch Henderson, singing at Take 6 and Denyce Graves at the Mann Center in Philadelphia, and again at the New Jersey Performing Arts Center. I even had to opportunity to tour with the choir in Atlanta, Georgia. Musically, I was exposed to a host of musical genres, such as spirituals, show tunes, musical theater, classical, pop, jazz, etc. And even though I could perform at a professional level, I was ill-equipped by way of music fundamentals (i.e., music history, musicianship/theory).

This has been a situation we encounter all too often in music education. There is a narrow range of skills considered to be "fundamental," and those tend to favor traditional private lessons-based knowledge not readily accessible to those whose experience had been mainly in ensemble-based settings where the repertoire is often outside of the Western canon.

In the fall of 2003, I started my first year of college at Westminster Choir College of Rider University. I saw the campus as a magical place where choral music existed. I was part of the college's chapel choir, the Westminster Jubilee Singers, and the Westminster Choir. . . . But my academic status suffered because I didn't speak enough of its mother tongue to guarantee my success (i.e., music fundamentals). I failed so badly at remedial musicianship courses, as well as other music courses that reinforced learning, that eventually I had to leave the school after three semesters. Needless to say, I was crushed! How could something I love so diligently not come easy by way of attending school? But was it (music and learning) on the top of my priority list? Was cultureshock (inner city black youth in a middle/upper class college town) attributed to my downfall? These are things I still ask myself to this day; I left the school full of shame and regret.

The "fundamentalist" perspective has permeated the curricula of music education and was the subject of what was the most "shameful and regrettable" [mis]representation of the profession in recent history. In a well-publicized May 2016 article in the *New York Times*, the then executive director of NAfME (the National Association for Music Education) was quoted as saying that the problem of diversifying the profession was due to his impression that "blacks and Latinos lack the keyboard skills needed for this field."[2] The article also reported comments regarding the lack of music theory training in the same populations, another unexamined trope considered to be "fundamental." Jeremy wrote his autobiography in September 2016, four months after he was presented this script for defining his perceived educational deficits.

Shortly thereafter (2005), I attended Bergen Community College and received a degree in Professional Studies. I took voice lessons on campus just for fun. I never learned any major repertoire because little by little, my love for singing began to fade away. Singing needed to become joyous again, and for a long time it hadn't.

In June 2005, my father died. I was nineteen years old. At this time, my father was in his seventies and my mother moved him back in. They had been apart for over ten years, but due to his failing health, she decided he was better in her care, which really meant our/my care. My mother couldn't deal with any funeral arrangements, so I planned everything. From what he wore in the casket, to the casket, pamphlets, flowers, etc. I was considered the smartest in the family, the "college boy." I was expected to hold it together.

I remember singing at his funeral. I had some friends from high school join me in singing "His Eyes Are on the Sparrow." I guess the reason why I decided to sing this song was because it was a staple at black funerals. But honestly, singing it wasn't some freeing experience. I suppose I was just going through

---

[2] Cooper, M. (2016, May 12). Music education group's leader departs after remarks on diversity. *New York Times*. https://www.nytimes.com/2016/05/13/arts/music/music-education-groups-leader-departs-after-remarks-on-diversity.html.

the motions. The real music, the real singing that washed my soul clean from heartbreak was the singing that happened late at night in my bedroom when I cried. I cried and sang myself to sleep to Luther Vandross's "Dance with my Father Again" for weeks.

This devastating trauma speaks to the complexity of Jeremy's narrative. He is negotiating many layers of identity, emanating from various developmental roles during this period: a son who has lost his father, a caretaker who assumes responsibility, a spiritual leader who provides soulful mediation for the grief-stricken—all while tending to his own loss.

In 2007, I enrolled at Ramapo College of New Jersey as a communications major. At this time, singing was nonexistent. The joy that I got from music left and my future career path was set. But in August of 2008, my mother passed away. There was no more career path for me, I had no future goals. Music wasn't in my life, and neither were the people who encouraged me to pursue it. Everything I knew and loved left my life. And so, I planned another funeral from top to bottom. All the responsibility was on me. I remember singing at her funeral. I again asked friends to help me sing "A Song for Mama," by Boyz2Men. But this time was different. When I began to sing this song, everyone in the room disappeared and it was only me and her. I was singing my goodbyes to one of the only women I would ever truly love. Singing my woes to a room full of friends and family was one of the hardest things I ever had to do.

Shortly thereafter, I dropped out of college and began working to sustain myself. I was putting in over seventy hours a week at jobs that paid horribly. I fell into a deep depression, started drinking alcohol and experimenting with drugs. . . . I lived exclusively on donated food from local pantries. I hit rock bottom. As a means to snap myself out of it, I remembered singing was the only thing that made me feel better. I decided to internet search a local choir and found the New Jersey Choral Society. Having the opportunity to perform alongside people who worked in other fields who come together to sing was so inspiring. And little by little, singing Mozart and Vaughan Williams, and the like, ignited my passion for singing once more. And when it was time, I would return back to school and attain a degree in music. In 2015, at the age of twenty-seven, I graduated Magna Cum Laude from Ramapo College with a Bachelor's of Arts degree in Music, with special concentrations in Voice Performance, Music Industry, and Music Studies. I was the assistant conductor of my college choir, president of my honor society. Music had become my saving grace.

Currently, I attend Teachers College for music and music education. I also teach second and third grade musicianship and choir for the Paterson Music Project, an El Sistema inspired program dedicated to using music as a vehicle of social justice. I never thought that my life could turn around in the way that it did. I never thought I would be in such a prestigious program at the master's level or that I would be cultivating the love of music in a child and providing them with the musical knowledge needed to speak the language at such a young age. I suppose my past experiences prepared me to become the teacher and role model my students need to see, especially because the school in which I teach is a half-block away from the home I lived in for over fifteen years. My students get to see someone who attended high school four blocks away in the city in which they live. I can be that person to cultivate the young minds of children to understand music and love playing an instrument or singing. From day one, I mattered. My life experiences have made me stronger. As a result, I feel that musically, I am the best version of myself, and my passion and purpose has grown exponentially due to my musical history.

We can see aspects of several narrative dimensions in this descriptive and honest self-reflection. There are elements of agency, such as doing an internet search to find a local choir when he knew he needed music in his life. Jeremy's process of meaning making is combined with his need for understanding the coherence he draws between his present and his past. His words reflect the redemptive sentiment found in many of the autobiographies: "*I suppose my past experiences prepared me to become the teacher and role model my students need to see. . . . From day one, I mattered.*"

Ruth (2016)

Unlike the first two narratives, Ruth's story reflects seventeen years of teaching in public schools—it is a story that she had most likely told previously in a variety of contexts. It is presented with attention to both informal and formal learning settings. It is also a story of heritage and hard work through which she reaped many rewards.

Music was a part of my set of languages as I was growing up. As far back as I can remember, there was English, Spanish, and music. English was the language my two older brothers and I used to speak to each other, and Spanish was the language we used to speak to our parents. Music was the language that gave my family meaningful connection. My mother made a living performing in a mariachi. She sang, and played guitar and vihuela, and continues to this day. I can remember hearing my mother sing and accompany herself on the guitar at any random time. After moving out of my home, I realized just what a gift it was, to have been immersed in music. Certainly, there is the value of having musical experiences as a child, but what was more meaningful was that this was how my mother expressed love and joy. My mother taught my brothers and me Spanish language children's songs from Mexico, and she would accompany us on the guitar while we sang "De Colores" at family parties. I enjoyed singing with my family, but as a shy child, I could not bring myself to sing alone in front of people. I always thought my mom showed great courage to sing on a stage in front of crowds of people in public spaces, and on television.

As my mother sang, in her interpretations, I could hear the feelings that she was expressing in her performances, and her musical peers would often comment to me as a child about how they enjoyed the heartfelt way that she sang with so much gusto. I grew up knowing Mexican folk music, known in Mexico as Ranchera. For a while, I didn't know there was music in other languages, since our radio and television were fixed on the same Spanish language radio stations, and it would be the same when we would go to Mexico to visit our relatives. I would hear Mariachi, Spanish pop, musica tropical (salsa, cha-cha-cha, merengue), cumbia, and norteño. I spent a lot of time in my elementary school years tagging along with my mother on her gigs, and hanging out in different performance venues, private events, and backstage in green rooms. She performed in many cultural events, so the education I got there was priceless. I saw the beauty of Mexican culture through music, dance, theater, and visual art. When I saw the ballet folklorico dancers, their movement and flowy dresses mesmerized me. At my request, my mother enrolled me in dance class to learn Mexican folk dances. I could feel myself express music through my body more easily than singing. I still felt so connected to the music, and so proud to have Mexican roots. I'm so thankful for this time in my life when my mother was my first music teacher, first and foremost, because these experiences taught me how much she loves me, and secondly because my elementary school did not have a music program. Throughout the time that my mother was my teacher, it always felt like fun, and the performance aspect of making music or dancing was never forced.

This rich musical environment was formative for Ruth. It inculcated her into a musical life, associated with positive emotion that established a foundation for future musical growth and enjoyment.

Going into sixth grade, I chose to play the clarinet. I was still too shy to sing in front of people, so choir was out of the picture. String orchestra seemed too nerdy, and I already had two bossy older brothers in band... who played... the trumpet. I think I would have liked to play the trumpet, but I was not about to go into the lion's den every day after school and hear it from my brothers about how I need to do things. So, I chose the clarinet ... sweet, small, portable, and NOT the trumpet. By my good fortune, my middle school did have an outstanding band program, and someone brand-new whose primary instrument was the clarinet would be my teacher. Her name is ReNee Nadeau. I found success quickly as a young musician as she taught me proper technique from the beginning, giving little chance for bad habits to form. She was encouraging, funny, and easy to approach. This was the beginning of our teacher/student relationship that evolved later into cooperating teacher/student teacher, mentor/mentee, colleagues, and finally lifelong friends. During the middle school years, the band would perform four times a year as an ensemble, and there were also honor band placement auditions, and solo and ensemble contests. I enjoyed any playing opportunity, and I most enjoyed playing in a woodwind quartet. ReNee organized us to rehearse and perform, and it was the first chamber music experience I had. I found the music to be so beautiful even in a small ensemble setting where my part could be easily heard with the exposed texture. I wished that I could have done more chamber music in that time, and that yearning never left as I continued over the years and into the present to collaborate with other musicians to rehearse and perform.

This attraction to playing in chamber ensembles was common among many of the autobiographies, and Ruth has identified the appeal of such activity. She writes, "*I found the music to be so beautiful even in a small ensemble setting where my part could be easily heard with the exposed texture.*" In these words, she offers a commentary on consequential participation: like Jeremy, she mattered. It is also notable how her relationship with ReNee

MUSICAL PATHWAYS   101

developed over time. This is a thread that runs through Ruth's narrative, as her relationships with several other teachers morphed easily into lifelong friendships.

> *High school band was where I felt an explosion of growth in my playing abilities. There were so many opportunities to rehearse, play, perform, and socialize within the band program. The upperclassmen took great responsibility in mentoring the underclassmen, the directors conducted the band as a whole, and the private instructors gave lessons to key musicians in the band. I learned most from those older students who were taking lessons, and then they shared what they learned with me. As a younger player, I was still expected to bring up my playing ability to match that of the older students. The most helpful friend I had was Scot Humes, and actually now he is Dr. Scot Humes, and is a Professor of Clarinet at University of Louisiana at Monroe. We are colleagues and friends, and I still call him for help. High school band was where I learned my voice as a solo musician. As I felt my expression, tone, and technique improving, I also felt myself maturing as a person, and being more insightful. I began studying out of etude books and solo repertoire including the Mozart Clarinet Concerto, works by Weber, and Stravinsky's Three Pieces for Clarinet Solo. I felt like maybe I was beginning to be good enough to consider it as a career. My self-doubt took me back and forth on this issue until my senior year, I earned a place in the Texas All-State Band, which is a three-month process of auditions across the state culminating in the selection of students to have the honor of performing in this band. It is the most rigorous audition process for students of this age that I've ever encountered. This was the break I was looking for that gave me affirmation that I could successfully study music and makes a living in the field.*

This major event in her life disrupted the feelings of self-doubt Ruth was feeling and renewed her sense of self-as-musician. It carried her on in the trajectory toward clarinet performance.

> *After a brief time at San Antonio College, I transferred to Texas State University where I studied clarinet with Dr. Pino who is the most influential teacher in my undergraduate education. Dr. Pino had a no-fault approach to teaching and gave me incredible freedom to choose my repertoire within reason and encouraged me by attending many of my performances. He organized a group of students to tour Switzerland, and our repertoire?*

Chamber music! We prepared music for string quartet plus clarinet for this tour including the Mozart Quintet and Brahms Quintet. It is still one of the highlights of my life, and I can't help but think about how much Dr. Pino really cared about us to put in so much work to take us all to Switzerland.

This return to chamber music brings a coherence to Ruth's narrative. She also acknowledges her teacher's care—a pedagogy that she adopted in her own teaching (personal communication).

Following student teaching, I taught high school and middle school band for two years, and then taught elementary music for fifteen years. While teaching elementary school, I earned a Master of Music degree from Texas A&M–Kingsville, where Dr. Nancy King Sanders was my clarinet teacher, graduate advisor, and taught many of the classes I took to complete this degree. She taught me to dream beyond my first inclination of what a big dream might be. There is so much more I could do.

This co-constructed dream for the future recalls her past and winning a place in the Texas All State Band. It is another disruption of negative scripts that disallow achievement. This teacher introduced unimagined possibilities—helping Ruth "to dream beyond [her] first inclination." This is a different form of disruption then has been previously discussed in this chapter: instead of interrupting an expected pathway to success, this disruption reveals an unexpected vision of the future.

The next phase of my musical learning came when I was hired onto the adjunct faculty at San Antonio College, and then I was accepted at the Imani Winds Chamber Music Festival. I had already been a fan of this wind quintet for many years; I considered them life-changing. I was so excited that they were launching a festival for wind quintet. At first, I was very scared, knowing that I would be auditioning alongside students from Juilliard, MSM, NYU, and other prestigious schools of music, and I did not have that kind of educational pedigree, just good old-fashioned hard work in the practice room. Upon being accepted, I was excited to learn that I would be performing a piece composed by the famous clarinetist, and one of my clarinet heroes, Paquito D'Rivera, and I would be performing it for him in a master class setting. I can still feel the magic that surrounded my body as his notes surrounded mine like a glove, and he added an improvised harmonized part over mine. The piece is called Preludio y Merengue.

After this festival, I formed my own wind quintet, Adelante Winds, and we programmed music by Latin American composers, and we performed in concert halls of various universities in Texas. This past June, the quintet came to be coached and performed at Imani Wind Chamber Music Festival. Since my coming to New York, they have continued to be active without me, and I have met some new friends in the city to make music with. I look forward to seeing what kinds of stories and recollections I would fill the next pages with.

Garnering a college teaching job and being chosen to play for/with a "clarinet hero" contributed to a sense of momentum that carried Ruth into the promise of her childhood and her "first teacher," whose lessons were delivered celebrating the performance of culturally relevant repertoire.

Claudia (2010)

Claudia's narrative provides an opportunity to revisit the two previous chapters though her rich descriptions of her childhood music experiences—she reminds us of the playful memories of early childhood and the epiphanies of discovery in middle childhood. Instead of many disruptions, this version of her story focuses on one major event that dramatically changes her trajectory and leads to a search for meaning that requires her agency.

When I was four years old, I've started playing the piano, following my dad's inspiration. The image of the two of us playing together, turning somersaults on the living room carpet, is still vivid in my mind, when suddenly my dad stopped spinning and, with a gorgeous smile, asked me, "Claudia, would you like to play the piano?" I don't recall ever having seen or heard a piano before, at least not consciously. What I do remember is my prompt answer "Yes, I'd love to!!!" returning his excitement with sparkling eyes and a smile. By chance, he had found a Japanese Suzuki piano teacher in my city—Perugia, Italy—and he couldn't have hoped for anything better than to realize the dream of his youth through his young daughter. Miss Setsuko Murata (now a lovely ninety years old) was primarily an opera singer, who had moved to Italy to master the language. It wasn't until much later that I discovered she was a very good friend of Dr. Suzuki during the dawning of the Suzuki Method around the world....

She had the most angelic voice and used to make me sing the melodies of the songs I was learning because, she said, "the way you listen and sing in your head creates your tone at the piano." She could barely speak Italian and she used to teach a lot by ear and through demonstration. A parent of one of my students has observed that my approach toward teaching mimics her playful attitude with a firm discipline. I also sing with my youngest students and teach by example, rather than words. As I stop to reflect on her now, I realize how much of her influence is present in my methods.

Claudia's narrative shows a strong coherence, as she draws together experiences from her learning into her teaching.

Her end-of-the-year recitals were quite famous in Perugia; I performed there six times, seeing [my name] moving down towards the most advanced part of the program, as I grew up. In one of my favorites, I performed "Für Elise" by Beethoven; it was quite an accomplishment to play such a piece for [child] barely nine years old, above all because through that piece I learned to use the pedal. And when a child discovers that this big instrument can make a smooth, intense, legato sound just by pushing down a small lever with her foot, she feels that she is a real pianist; this discovery was overwhelming!

This moment of clarity regarding her identification as a musician comes early for Claudia. She attributes much of this to her father's commitment.

However, what kept me with her for six years . . . [was] my dad with his patience and devotion to music and me. We used to practice together at the piano everyday throughout my elementary school years. I have a great sense of gratitude for my dad because I've learned how to love piano through his love for my instrument. His studio, with a little lamp on the piano, was our world. During this time, playing the piano meant just spending more time with my daddy, laughing at each other's mistakes, repeating the same section one hundred times and negotiating for less if it was without mistakes, or just playing some four hands pieces. Our favorites were without a doubt, the "Four Hands Pieces" by Diabelli. Much of my approach with children is about re-creating the magical time and intimate joy that my father created with me. I believe that my role as a teacher is all about helping children fall in love with their instrument.

When I turned ten, my teacher suggested that I audition for the conservatory, where I could study on scholarship with very great professors. Certainly, my musical training took off toward a more serious and demanding path. . . . My time at the conservatory very quickly became the most demanding and busy years of my entire life: I always felt high expectations from professors and consequently from family and friends. For the nature of the institution as it's conceived in Italy, I could attend the conservatory at the same time as my regular high school, whereas I had spent my middle school years in a special school just for students admitted to the music program. I refer to this as the time of "studio matto e disperatissimo," which in Italy means literally "The most crazy and despaired study." It's a very common expression in Italian to highlight situations of overwhelming work which can threaten personal health and well-being. I used to spend four or five hours a day in my practice room, in addition to completing my regular schoolwork. Emotionally, I was in love with my instrument and, as with any love story, I could have given my life for music. I felt I could change the world by just playing my piano with such energy, concentration and heart-blood engagement. . . .

However, my continuous study undermined an already quite fragile physical constitution, and after my graduation at nineteen years old, I fell ill. Consequently, my studies at University of Perugia in Italian Literature (my major was History of Music) experienced a sudden setback and the pattern of me being an exemplary student was miserably broken. I became angry at myself for being sick. I was mad because while I was recovering, I lost all of my musical connections and precious time of my youth. Moreover, on a larger scale, I faced the reality of being just a pianist among enormous quantities of great pianists. I felt unsuccessful and hopeless.

Such a significant disruption stops the trajectory in its directional course, leaving the individual to reassess and retool a musical life.

During this period, I learned how hard and competitive a musical career can be; hence I often considered other job options for my life. Although, relentlessly and without fail, everything took me back to music: my church choir (a young, informal setting all about having fun with music), some good friends interested in learning piano, and an overall a sort of musical aura that made me the "musical expert" in my own community of family and friends. I wanted to push music away and I felt it was like a gravitational force, drawing me back, anywhere and all the time.

Many of us have learned about musical meaning through our pedagogical lens. Claudia was no exception.

In the meantime, I had started teaching piano and early childhood music classes. Unfortunately, the traditional way of teaching learned at the conservatory didn't fit my sensitivity or match the joy I experienced with Miss Murata. I often felt like a "fish out of water" compared to my colleagues and did not have tools to support my concept of teaching. I was deeply frustrated.

After significant personal struggle, Miss Murata advised me to attend the Suzuki teacher training in London as the best way to solve my self-perceived inadequacy as a teacher. That course opened my eyes and provided me with the tools I needed as well as the "philosophy" of teaching I've always felt true for me.

During the same time, I started meeting with a spiritual friend, a very inspirational wise nun (Sister Luisella) who helped me to find my own unique voice in music. With her perceptive guidance and the conceptual setting of the Suzuki philosophy, I realized that I could really touch people's hearts and shape their characters through music. In this sense, my piano playing became an open window for me to explore what is inexpressible in words but can't be left unsaid. Through Dr. Suzuki, I've learned that "Having great ability means having a deep and great ability of the heart" and that if "I really would like to be more talented, I should make my heart more talented."

This shift in purpose to a talented heart came with a newfound respect for the impact of a life spent teaching music. Such a shift, although couched in different words, was a common experience for many of the autobiographers.

Clara, Jeremy, Ruth, and Claudia each had a different arc to their storied narrative. For Clara, it was a series of peaks and valleys, which were navigated with the support of parents, teachers, and peers. For Jeremy, circumstances out of his control created intense highs and lows, mediated, in part, by his attunement to the affordances that music provided. For Ruth, it was a steady movement through time, punctuated by affirming experiences that provided impetus for becoming, facilitating choices and direction. For Claudia, the narrative shape comprised a single devastating disruption requiring a redefinition of musical self, transforming hopelessness into flourishing through the power of past and present relationships and future possibility.

Teaching Narratives and Generativity

After I pursued my master's degree at Peabody, I thought about my career in music. I wanted to share my joy of music with other people. I wanted to inspire people the way my teacher [inspired] me. I wanted to let people know how great music is. I wanted to share my great [moments] of music. . . . I wanted to do those things in a direct way. After I pondered the idea, I came up with the answer. That was: "teaching music." (Claire, 1999)

In his analyses of autobiographical writing, McAdams (2015) discusses the significance of generativity, that is, being motivated to contribute to the well-being of future generations. He names parenting and teaching as two roles that are characteristically generative, as they are specifically responsible for children's learning and preparedness for the future. It turns out that musical parenting contributes to future generations. In a national survey of new parents (Custodero & Johnson Green, 2003), we found that the strongest predictor of whether a parent would sing to their baby was if they remembered being sung to. This was true for many students who wrote about how their memories of their own teachers influenced their approach to music education—like Claire, they spoke of the joy which came from sharing their love of music with others.

For Ari, the journey to music educator was predicated on the development of his own musicianship. His language suggests generativity: he writes of "passing on" his knowledge and wanting to "show the next generation how to climb this mountain." In the narrative below, he shares how his motivation for teaching evolved from extrinsic financial goals to intrinsic meaningful rewards:

I knew that I would have to find a way to make money in order to support myself. I turned once again to private teaching. Through a company that matched piano teachers to students in their area, I accumulated a tidy little studio of eager young musicians. It was at this point that a little nugget of realization began to form in the back of my mind. I was enjoying what I had originally intended to be merely a for-profit endeavor, and I was especially gratified when a student asked me to help him learn "Let It Be"; in a few weeks he was slamming C–Am–G–F and belting it out. I see now that I was too selfishly deep into my goal of supporting myself through playing alone to fully embrace this budding love of teaching, but there it stayed, biding its time. As I established myself in Columbus, I found a wealth of musical mentors and collaborators across a broad spectrum of genres and backgrounds. With a vocalist classmate and her Brazilian beau, we started a group that played the energetic, danceable pop of Brazil. Through that band's work, I met a bassist from Peru who recruited me for a band that fused rhythms from his country with Santana-style guitar heroics. I spent thousands of joyous hours with jazz groups of every stripe. I joined a bar band that specialized in lithe, bluesy soul, playing hits by Al Green, Prince, and interpreting a host of other pop standards. This time in my life was one of great happiness and fulfillment, and it also helped me find myself as a person—now I could call myself a musician and really mean it. Now I could truly pass on my knowledge. Why do I want to teach music? Quite simply, it is because I love what music has done for me, and I want to show the next generation how to climb this mountain. The view is spectacular. (Ari, 2013)

Motivation researchers have found that monetizing an intrinsically rewarding activity can have a negative effect on the joy experienced in that activity (Deci & Flaste, 1996). In Ari's narrative, the opposite occurred, suggesting that music making may be resilient to the motivational effects of monetary promise.

In the following excerpt, violinist Kokoe compares her memory of a transformational experience she had as a young performer playing in an ensemble, with a similar experience she facilitated for her students. (The bold font is from her original document.)

Age 14: I still can close my eyes and remember how I felt when we performed this piece in Carnegie Hall. I remember stepping onto the stage and feeling intense emotions of excitement. I felt how vast and extraordinary the hall was and how honored I felt to step onto this stage that so many great virtuosos had performed on. I recall the stillness and silence before the conductor cued us to start and feeling the intensity of the beating timpani as we played our first note. I could not believe how incredible we sounded, **living and feeling the music in every fiber of my being**, *and creating an unforgettable musical memory.*

*Age 30: Last November, the school where I teach was invited by WQXR, NY Public Radio, to perform at their most prestigious annual gala event. We were asked to select only five students to perform and decided to play Canon in D by Pachelbel. We stepped on stage after they shared with the audience the documentary trailer of the film we are featured in, and the ballroom was packed, and the energy was high. I do not usually get nervous, but I suddenly felt my heart beating rapidly and I just took one look at my students whom I've known since they were ages five–six and felt a surge of excitement and happiness. It was as if I was momentarily brought back and saw them as young children and then immediately as the young adults they have grown into and I just smiled to myself and took a deep breath. All five of my students had their eyes on me, the spotlight shown on their lovely faces, and they smiled back, and we began. This performance nearly brought me to tears **because I could feel their focus and concentration and it felt like we had taken a leap forward together; we were simply enjoying ourselves, listening to one another, and ultimately making music**. It was our most heartfelt performance and I was so proud of my students. It is incredible to have these experiences that live on in my memory and how I recall certain events that have shaped my life; and now how I am giving my students the opportunity and tools to experience unforgettable musical memories. (Kokoe, 2016)*

Kokoe draws together her past with her present in a celebration of coherence of her student musician and music teacher stories. She recognizes the meaning in the immersive quality of musical performance, especially powerful in communion with others. This dimension of her narrative recalls Jeremy's description of singing at his mother's funeral ("*everyone in the room disappeared and it was only me and her*") and Ruth's duet with Paquito D'Rivera ("*I can still feel the magic that surrounded my body as his notes surrounded mine like a glove*"). It may be that capacity for deep engagement in music making is another idiosyncratic quality that defines our experiences.

What is really driving these narratives of impassioned music teaching, and the acknowledgment of rewards of sharing the learners' discovery? It is because we are musical beings, whose humanity is modeled in the communicative, expressive, and comfort of musical experience: to share this is to share our humanity. Teachers like Kokoe get to relive the thrill of their early experiences of belonging and discovery, expanding the concept of generativity to include the regeneration of self through their work with students.

Elise has figured it out:

I am still struggling a bit to digest and find peace with my experience in the conservatory setting. One reason that I love to work with young kids and children with special needs is that they aren't in that space. They likely aren't thinking of their music making in the context of "Am I really good enough?" or "Am I only doing this because I'm good at it?" They are more easily able to experience the music making for what it is in the moment. It is a gift to help a child find joy and gain insight through music and an important reminder as to why I love music. (Elise, 2015)

The answer comes from the children.

6
Encounters with Children
Lessons on Mutuality and Possibility

The Legacy of Children

In the preceding three chapters, I have examined the influences of childhood memories on our current circumstances and values. Looking at our own histories provides evidence for a coherent framework that can identify who we are and suggest possibilities for who we will become. In this chapter, I turn the kaleidoscope to another source of light: the legacy of our encounters with children.

I've worked with many professional musicians to help them find authentic ways to be musical with young children. In an interview with Marco, a jazz drummer, he shared, "What I like about kids is that they have an ancestral way to relate. I think that they can read and see a lot of what we forgot." This sense of children as representative of our heritage, and the idea that they have a valuable naiveté and an unfettered read on the world has been noted in the teaching of spiritual leaders such as Lao Tzu (Taoism)[1] and Jesus (Christianity),[2] and scholars like Edith Cobb. Questions about the child that exists in each of us, and what insight and clarity children may bring to our attention, have been part of human inquiry for thousands of years—there is much to be learned from continuing the exploration.

We are vulnerable to the enticing presence of children. Riding on the subway, there are few experiences that bring more moments of collective delight than the shared observation of a child who is engaging in musical play—spontaneously singing or moving rhythmically or acting out a dramatic episode with a toy or a friend. There is recognition from all observers

---

[1] Lao-Tzu has asked his followers: "Can you center your energy, be soft, tender and so learn to be a baby?" (p. 10).

[2] In the biblical book of Matthew, chapter 18, verses 1–3, we find this reference: "At that time the disciples came to Jesus, saying, 'Who is the greatest in the kingdom of heaven?' And calling to him a child, he put him in the midst of them and said, 'Truly, I say to you, unless you turn and become like children, you will never enter the kingdom of heaven.'"

that what they are witnessing is a product of unbridled imagination in response to an environment that provided the necessary affordances (Gibson, 1977) such as billboards with pictures or recognizable symbols. Systematic observations confirmed this with reports of one child breaking out in a rendition of "The ABC Song" in response to seeing the letters posted for the subway lines, and another, who started improvising a song about a dog as he looked at a photo of one on a poster (Custodero, Calì, & Diaz Donoso, 2016).

Structures of the train also invite much playful engagement—the bells sounding when the train is preparing to leave the station are ripe for vocal imitation, the floor-to-ceiling poles are interesting to twirl around and feel the inertia of a contoured phrase, and the bench seats provide a perch from which one can peer out the windows into the darkness, giving a sense of being alone and private. This arrangement often generates self-soothing in the form of quiet humming and singing. As I notice these behaviors, I make eye contact with my fellow adult passengers, communicating that we have just seen something that has momentarily taken us from the mundane to the sublime.

What is it that draws us to these actions by children? I return to the idea of mutuality—of adults seeing something as familiar, recognizing it as something they have experienced or have wanted to experience sometime in their lives. It allows us to see ourselves in one another, to view children as unfiltered representations of humanity. Like the concept of kinship, it brings a sense of belonging to a group of people who share a common experience.

The recognition of the adult self in children can elicit different types of responses from enchantment to regret, from delight to melancholy to indifference. However, it has been my experience that in recounting our feelings about these observations, the vocabulary used to describe what we have encountered is limited and based on assumptions about the observed, without considering the positioning of the observer. The descriptor I have most often heard for our appreciation of children is "cute," a generic reference to the "look" of what we see, an objectification, void of any deeper meaning. If Wittgenstein (1968) was correct, and the limits of our language do reflect the limits of our mind, then we must work to adopt a more descriptive repertoire to fully comprehend the legacy of children.

Leonard Bernstein was sensitive to this simplistic adult treatment of children and imagined the child's concomitant response. In 1943 he published *I Hate Music! A Cycle of 5 Kid's Songs for Soprano and Piano* for which he wrote both words and music. The fifth song, "I'm a Person Too," is particularly pertinent here:

> I just found out today, that I'm a person too, like you: I like balloons; lots of people like balloons: But ev'ryone says "Isn't she cute? She likes balloons!" I'm a person too, like you! I like things that ev'ryone likes: I like soft things and movies and horses and warm things and red things: don't you? I have lots of thoughts; like what's behind the sky; and what's behind what's behind the sky: But ev'ryone says, "Isn't she sweet? She wants to know ev'rything!" Don't you? Of course, I am very young to be saying all these things in front of so many people like you: But I'm a person too! Though I'm only 10 years old; I'm a person too, like you.

Through these lyrics, Bernstein is demonstrating an empathetic understanding of children's struggles to be treated respectfully. In the following pages, I examine enchantment as a framework to explain what is behind our default description of "cute" and suggest possible alternatives to describe our encounters with children. I am interested in how we learn from children's presence in our lives, and how out interactions affect the values, mood, and musicality of adults.

Observers and Observed: Embodied, Enchanted, and Compassionate

As we read in Chapter 3, parents and other caregivers use music with infants—to calm and soothe them, to entertain them, and to accompany everyday routines. We sing lullabies specific to our cultural identities; we also create music for the moment, to provide a soundtrack to our daily activity. We do this because babies are receptive to our music making, engaged by tunes and rhythms that come from us, their culture bearers. Sharing our voices is how we bring them into our circle of belonging: they provide feedback that invites our sustained engagement. In studies of musical parenting, researchers have found parents to have a natural tendency to share musical experiences with their infants and young children (e.g., Custodero & Johnson-Green, 2003, 2008; Illari, 2005, Koops, 2019). When infants respond to our musical cues, they join with us, mimicking our musical sounds in their vocalizations, and we in turn reciprocate, in a co-constructed musical dialogue.

In the spirit of interdisciplinarity that permeates this book, I review several theories that, in combination provide a broad canvas for thinking about musical encounters between adult and child partners. Communicative Musicality (Malloch and Trevarthen, 2009) discussed elsewhere in the book, is based on the shared motive pulse and identified by the synchronicity of vocalizations between parent and infant. Situating experience in listening, communicative musicality indicates our need to join with one another, trying to emulate what we hear. Calì (2015, 2020) has expanded the theory to include older children in the family context; her work acknowledges specific, idiosyncratic contributions from each member that define the musical life of the sound group. The original and expanded versions of communicative musicality put forth strong evidence for an intersubjective framework for explaining and enhancing most adult-child partnerships, including teacher-student. Below, I present three related lenses through which to view the dialogue between self and other.

Baby's Darwin and Embodied Participation

In a landmark article, Conrad (1998) provides a comparative analysis of Charles Darwin's diary and his published scientific report on observations of his own infant's development. The report, published thirty-seven years after the diary was completed, was emotionally distanced, void of any mention of the relationship between the observer and the observed—it was "scientifically objective." The diary, however, told a different story, one that showed a development of mutual recognition between Darwin and his baby. In the public version, the scientist assumed the role of "detached observer"; in the diary version, the adult-as-partner became an "embodied participant" (p. 16).

In reading through the diary documentation, Conrad noted that the need for a dynamic, subjective connection was expressed by both Darwin and his infant son—the observer and the observed. What seemed to motivate the active and personal responses was Darwin's awareness of the child being aware of him: the mutuality of the exchange was the key to unlocking his detachment and opening the door to emotional and responsive interaction and knowledge production. The experience of being seen is a powerful motivator for communication.

There was a progression Conrad found in the diary that began with Darwin referencing his child as "it," a practice that was replaced within a few months with the use of personal pronouns and eventually, loving nicknames. Based on her examination, she suggests a taxonomy of mutual recognition, which spanned the ages of 4.5 months to 32 months:

- Reciprocal Action
- Action in Relation to Recognized Other
- Recognition of Self in Other and Other in Self
- Reciprocal Observation
- Elaboration of Self in Relation to Other and Other in Relation to Self

Mutual recognition can be used to explain the act of singing a lullaby when both parent and child are recognizing and trusting the intention of the other in relation to self. Ensemble experiences can be significant when the individual musicians recognize and respond to each other's intentions. Mutual recognition is also present in stories of teaching and learning when both student and teacher can experience together the aesthetic exuberance of creating music. Tanya's story comes to mind, especially her recollection of performing with her teacher in a band accompanying the school musical: *"At that moment, I realized that the notes created by our essence had transformed into chords that carried us and the audience into a utopia of music."* Tanya's experience of mutual recognition was multilayered in that it included both fellow musicians and audience.

Music provides a privileged setting for mutual recognition, as it is responsive to the implicit understandings that originate in sound rather than linguistics. It fits with Johnson's (2007) description of embodiment and its beginnings in infancy: "body-based intersubjectivity—our being with others via bodily suggestion, gesture, imitation and interaction—is constitutive of our very identity from our earliest days, and it is the birthplace of meaning" (p. 51). Our experiences are underscored as we are physically and emotionally moved by music because we see our responses in the bodies of others. We also recognize the novelty or familiarity of a tune or rhythmic pattern and share the associations. Given this special status of musical experience—its embodied qualities, its capacity to provoke mutual recognition, and its provision of implicit understanding—it follows that adults turn to children as exemplars of attunement to meaning.

Enchantment and Compassionate Intelligence as Responses to Children

As was the case with Darwin, our encounters with young children produce an unmasking of the objective, distantly academic, and controlled persona, revealing a vulnerability to surprise and delight. This is the effect of being open to mutuality—we are surprised to hear an infant echo a sound we make or see a toddler bouncing up and down to our favorite rock anthem because these are activities in which we engage. We don't expect to see ourselves in children so young, and we are emotionally moved by it. Such a response may perhaps best be described as enchantment, which, as Bennett (2001) writes, is "to be struck and shaken by the extraordinary that lives amid the familiar and every day" (p. 4). I believe this may be what the observers of young children who use the word "cute" are experiencing.

Bennett also contends that enchantment allows us to briefly experience the response to the world we had as children. She writes: "The overall effect of enchantment is a mood of fullness, plentitude or liveliness, a sense of having one's nerves or circulation, or concentration powers tuned up or recharged—a shot in the arm, a fleeting return to childlike excitement about life" (p. 5). Like Conrad, she is mindful of the corporeal aspects of the experience and the need for embodied, sympathetic understanding of the other.

In the first chapter of this book, I discussed the relationships between music, time, and space and the countermotions that create dynamism in our experience. Enchantment is a feeling that may be conjured by that dynamism, as we are "simultaneously transfixed by wonder and transported by sense, to be both caught up and carried away" (Bennett, 2001, p. 5). Being transported is a countermotion to being transfixed, and these two forces in simultaneity suggest a vibrant tension that is reflected in the description of enchantment above. Borrowing from Phillip Fisher (1998), Bennett describes such experiences as "moments of pure presence," when all of our energies converge in an exhilarating sensory rush of implicit understanding. Being with young children can incite these feelings.

Bennett makes a strong argument for the role of enchantment in enacting ethical practices. She writes:

> Enchantment is a feeling of being connected in an affirmative way to existence; it is to be under the momentary impression that the natural and

cultural worlds *offer gifts* and, in doing so, remind us that it is good to be alive. This sense of fullness ... encourages the finite human animal, in turn, to give away some of its own time and effort on behalf of other creatures. (p. 156)

Enchantment shares many traits with Cobb's (1977) concept of "compassionate intelligence," which honors our "nature to nurture." While proposing that we all carry the potential to be destructive, she offers hope that such potential is mediated by our awareness of the child's sense of wonder and an acknowledgment of not knowing, which leads to "a special type of humility infused with joy" (p. 107). She traces compassionate intelligence to the reciprocity of the parent-child relationship and advocates for capitalizing on the enchantment that generates the impulse to nurture.

Becoming aware of children's music making, as is described above in the subways or at home, in a classroom, or on the playground, calls us to honor the extraordinary that exists in our otherwise disenchanted world. It is Bennett's contention that by dismissing the potential for enchantment, we are left with the disenchantment script, which cannot sustain the needed attention to work toward societal good. She purports that "presumptive generosity, as well as the will to social justice, are sustained by periodic bouts of being enamored with existence" (p. 12). The words of Cobb and Bennett suggest that attending to children's musical invitations and responses provide moments of sustenance to carry on, a reminder of our affiliative connections to music and to others. To examine the possibilities of these phenomena, I present a case study of musicians and infants, and their experiences of mutual recognition, enchantment, and compassion in the creation and performance of an opera.

BambinO: A Case Study of an Opera Composed and Performed for Infants

Background

When we first think of music for babies, we don't think of a live opera performance, given the exaggerated emotional tone and stylized adult interpretation of story. However, in 2016 the Scottish Opera, located in Glasgow, felt compelled to engage with this challenge and commissioned a forty-minute interactive opera for six-to-eighteen-month-olds, *BambinO*. They organized a touring company complete with set, props, stage manager, two singers (soprano and baritone), and two instrumentalists (cellist and percussionist). Designed to be performed for and with babies, *BambinO* presents a unique example of an operatic production comprising multiple layers of collaboration and response that contributed to an authentic and relevant experience for performers and audiences alike.

In the spring of 2018, *BambinO* came to New York City (see Figure 6.1). The troupe performed ten shows for audiences of twenty-four parent (or caregiver) and infant pairs; reservations were needed, but there was no charge for the tickets. Performances took place on the stage floor of a recital hall in the Metropolitan Opera House (MET), and the set consisted of a large circular area bounded by a small, raised platform on which the instrumentalists perched, with a few rows of benches and chairs for the adults on the opposite side. Between those boundaries was a soft large rug on which was placed a sea of soft pillows meant to be an inviting and safe environment for infants, available for climbing or hiding or resting or jumping.

Additional sensitivity to the young audience included attentiveness to multimodal learning using manipulatives such as small chirping cloth birds that the infants could hold and move. Parents were available for whatever the child needed—a lap on which to sit, a nod of permission to approach the singer, or someone to share the humor of the baritone making faces. In line with research on children's development, attachment to their adults is crucially important to infants' feelings of safety in new environments (Mikulincer, Shaver, & Pereg, 2003).

Two colleagues, Nita Baxani and Susan Recchia, and I were invited by the MET to do research on the project. We collected field notes during performances, video of five presentations, as well as interviews and focus groups with the composer, director, stage manager, instrumentalists, and singers to document their ideas and reflections about doing opera with babies. Everyone involved with the program was energized by this work with infants—from our discussions, it was clear that they were embracing the challenge of introducing a musical style that they loved to these young listeners.

ENCOUNTERS WITH CHILDREN   119

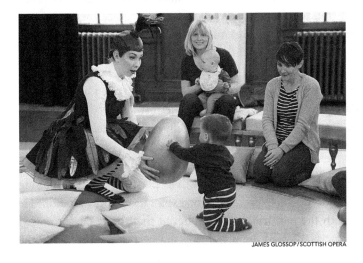

Figure 6.1 *BambinO* at the Metropolitan Opera

Composing with Infants in Mind

In developing the musical content for the opera, the composer, Lliam Paterson, drew from a variety of sources and took on different roles in the process of educating himself about his new audience and their interests. One role was that of musician, in which he drew upon his knowledge and expertise to share a cultural heritage. The composer's choice to score a variety of live instruments performed by a professional cellist and percussionist, in addition to opera singers who used their full voice and range as well as acting abilities, contributed to the musical authenticity of the piece. Paterson's musical background served to ensure that operatic conventions were included—he quoted snippets of several familiar pieces, such as the bird duet from Mozart's *The Magic Flute*. In "Notes from the Composer" from the *BambinO* printed score, he writes:

> This work is unequivocally an opera aimed at the most open of ears. The essence of Baroque, Mozartian, Bel Canto, Modernist, and even Minimalist opera makes an appearance, all within a playfully experimental piece which reflects my own voice as a composer too.

Through including so many operatic styles in a "playful" way, he is mining the legacy of children—their proclivity for exploration and imitation. He also connects with the performers who believed that the uncompromised quality of their parts allowed them to bring the best of themselves to the performances.

In addition to his musical expertise, Paterson also took on the role of researcher, investigating what developmental psychology could tell him about this new audience. He read academic literature, including one particularly thought-provoking area of research on universal baby language. He incorporated these infant speech patterns and vocalizations in the libretto.[3]

Paterson also took a research approach in his composing by collecting observational data, again in his "Notes from the Composer":

> There was a fantastic opportunity to carry out our own first-hand research when the workshops week culminated in an audience of 10 babies and their mothers observing our experiments! Their feedback (both the more immediate responses of the babies and the thought-through feedback of the parents) has been invaluable shaping the work.

Here we also see a third role as he takes up the position of collaborator, attending to the feedback from infants and parents—his intended

---

[3] Paterson studied the "Dunstan baby language," which purports to have identified five sounds that all infants used across cultures to communicate with adults and each other. https://www.dunstanbaby.com.

audience. The workshops he mentions were key to this project. Led by Phelim McDermott, the director of the opera, a group of singers and musicians along with the composer met for a week and experimented with sound and movement. This collaborative approach to creating a piece engendered a sense of investment and ownership of the project that gave the performers confidence. In the presentation of the opera, they knew the material well; it had been organically conceived with their participation, so they had enough certainty about the musical intention to be open and take risks when the infants' actions required a new response. They recalled the workshops with gratitude and joy, as can be seen in this excerpt from their focus group interview:

COMPOSER: It was really interesting because we had that sort of . . . personal and emotional bonding process during the workshop week in December 2016. So, when I turned up for the workshops with these guys, so . . . the current cast was part of the workshop group of the performers that were there, so I was sort of getting to know everyone on an emotional, personal level, and then also what their playing was like and then I was directly responding, writing the opera—

CELLIST: The Exploration aria where Tim (the Baritone) goes "broooop" (ascending slide and then descending). That started off with "here's a bunch of ideas" and then we kind of improvised it and then we wrote it down.

COMPOSER: And that actually wasn't altered at the end of the workshop in the final score.

BARITONE: No, it went straight in there. Yeah, yeah, yeah.

CELLIST: Which is quite nice.

COMPOSER: Yeah, but I think that's really an important part of creating a piece like this because you have to, and you guys are all so wonderful at doing this, but because you have to respond to your audience in such a unique way and like very quickly, that it's like it was important to write music that, I guess, chimed with you all on a personal level.

BARITONE: The ownership of us as a group of performers, that is really great for that reason.

A minute later, he adds:

The confidence we have because we created it together, to take it back to the babies that's what gives us the confidence to be so flexible and malleable and interactional with the kids, I think.

The collaborative spirit in the making of this opera extended into its performance—in many ways this model of democratic participation suggests mutual recognition, starting with the composer and musicians. Being invited into the creation of the work primed the singers and instrumentalists for listening and responding to cues from their audience.

Performing with Children in Mind

The four musicians were aware of the need to be responsive to their audience. The percussionist, Stuart, was especially conscious of the collaborative nature of the compositional process and its effect on the performances.

> Percussionist: Yes, I think that's the most important thing and I think... that it's a credit to the music and what Lliam's done.... I can mold what I'm doing with the music sometimes whether that's dynamically or speed or things like that. The audience members dictate what's happening in our performance, [we do this] to give them more enjoyment. So, I mean, for instance, ... if there is a baby being brought over to my side, I'm not going to maybe hit things as hard, or maybe if they're really enjoying it, I might hit it harder.

Here, Stuart is an embodied participant, living in the present moment, attuned to his audience. He attributes that to the collaborative engagement with his fellow musicians:

> So, you're reacting to them and the music and the nature of what we've learned to do with each other. It means that we can do that well, and it makes the performance and the enjoyment of the performance better. But what we've learned maybe through doing it so much is that you have to revel in what they dictate us to do. You can't [think], "Oh, why are they clapping? Because I'm trying to play in 5/8; you [babies] can't do that." You just enjoy it and you're almost like music making with them because, you know, that's what we thought of right from the start—they're the show. So again, ... Lliam's sort of worked his magic [with us] ... [and it] works as an organic process between us and the audience, that we got to engage with them.

"They're the show." It feels as though Stuart has developed an enchantment script as a way to maximize the experience for both himself and the audience. He emphasizes this later in the focus group:

> But I think engaging with one is sometimes really beautiful. I actually just happened to have that happen in the last show. It was quite near the end. I can't remember what he got drawn in to but he was looking right at me and so maybe—so it must have been after Tim's flying off because I remember then I picked up the bird and he was smiling, and he was just mesmerized and so happy to see what I was going to do next; and I think it was really good to revel in that moment for me just to say, okay I'm going to perform for you right now and not—and focus it for him or her at that moment rather than have it as a bigger thing and you can just bring it right in for him.

Stuart has described a "moment of pure presence" where he experiences the feeling of plentitude, which infants can provide. Below, he brings in the emotional component of the interactions:

> It goes back to . . . that interactive thing, so I think it's because we're doing our job so well as actors, then what happens in the performance dictates how we act. So, if something happens like sometimes what's happening musically and what happens with someone in the audience, and it might also be something that's going on in your head at that time. For me personally then and if I get emotional and you think you could almost cry, you go with it, or I do at least. And I might look at the children and be emotional with them and I think you can't underestimate that they can feel that a full live human [who is] being emotional with them.

"Circles of Wonderfulness"

Stuart describes these emotionally imbued moments and infers a feeling of enchantment in the ways in which he is both transfixed by an emotionally intense experience and transported into a temporary mindset that leaves the worries and everyday challenges behind, allowing him to "revel in the moment."

PERCUSSIONIST: But it's a real thing, it's not a joke. I've definitely had moments in the show when you feel emotional that you could almost cry with them, and then you've created something really beautiful and there might be other things that are going on with you that morning or after the show and then you're allowed to revel in that moment that—it happened to me this week so it's a real thing.

Susan, an infant specialist and leader of our research team, responds to him, in an affirming dialogue:

SUSAN: It's very powerful. And babies do have this way of . . >
PERCUSSIONIST: Yeah!
SUSAN: You know, it's the connection
BARITONE: So honest!
PERCUSSIONIST: Yeah!
SUSAN: It's authentic.
PERCUSSIONIST: Yeah, that's right! There's not that barrier there that we adults put up, that's right, and that is an organic [experience] that we can have with them and enjoy . . . that's right.
SUSAN: They bring it out in us because that's what they are. They're in the moment.
PERCUSSIONIST: Yes.

In our interview with Phelim McDermott, the director, he mentioned that what has been most fascinating for him are the intimate moments he has observed between parent, child, and performer. Specifically, he talked about the options of watching the opera itself, the babies enjoying the opera, and the parents watching the babies enjoying the opera. In describing the simultaneous presence of those perspectives, he used the metaphor of an electronic circuit board all lit up. McDermott credits Paterson's scoring for the creation of "holding spaces" from which to observe others' responses, allowing time in the structure of the opera to advantage these openings for mutual recognition. Tim, the Baritone, alluded to these opportunities for experiencing multiple perspectives:

I also like that, you know, [we use] that kind of Disney formula that they make a film for children but it's also—there are little things for adults there too. It's such a circle of wonderfulness because you make the parents happy, you make the kids happy.

These communicative expressions, social behaviors, and responsive interactions that the performance engendered for infants and their caregivers were also reciprocally experienced by the singers and instrumentalists. The nature of this work was unique for all the artists, particularly with the need for ongoing improvisation as they worked so directly and interpersonally with the babies. This experience seems to have had an impact on their overall approach to their work as teachers, learners, and performers.

Enchanted by Surprise: The Rewards of Letting Go

The performers wanted to share moments of surprise and delight they had experienced with the children and with each other. Tim recalled being vulnerable in a scene in which he is hidden under an assortment of pillows in anticipation of "hatching" from the egg:

BARITONE: For me, being under all those pillows, [it often happens that] you get ones who want to take me out. And I remember lying there and I am completely helpless under there and there's nothing I can do. They just climb on me... they were hitting me with the pillows. And then there was this really funny one, they [removed] one perfectly [placed] in front of my face. You know, it looks like a giant baby coming at you, it's really interesting (laughter).

SOPRANO: Oh, I loved the, there was a little girl who absolutely adored Laura's [cello] playing. And she does these great glissandi that [go] "wooop" (upward inflection) and every time she did this gliss [the child] sat right in front of her and she absolutely giggled—had a giggle fit—that was brilliant. (laughter) They just love it because it sounds like, I don't know, "mmm" (upward inflection) something, like a rude noise maybe. I love it and she was properly giggling, that was really funny.

These responses to action-based, embodied interactions with infants reflect the enchantment script and an appreciation for what children bring to our view of the world. Members of this *BambinO* opera troupe provide a model of Cobb's compassionate intelligence, as they seek out goodness in the infants and accept the goodness in themselves. This work also seems to encourage both humility and confidence in the performers.

SOPRANO: For me in reply to your questions, well I feel like because I graduate this summer so I'm at quite at the beginning of my career in opera—fingers crossed. So, for me doing these performances has given me so much confidence in myself and confidence in learning that when you're in a troupe, when you're part of a team, the magic is in the ensemble. And the show is made by people, not just one person who's up on that stage giving an aria.

CELLIST: It's chamber music.

SOPRANO: Yeah, but even with a huge orchestra, you can't, you can't make magic alone. It's a show and all of it comes together and I kind of thought if I can sing in front of babies who might cry, then I can sing my audition in front of grumpy old men or . . . (laughter)

BARITONE: Phelim says that this will prepare us for any performance ever, ever again. It's kind of true . . . what I feel good about this project is that it would probably give me like "I could probably do anything." I'd be happy to do anything important because we've had to . . .

SOPRANO: We wanted to. We've learned to enjoy the crazy and like know that actually that's not a crazy thing to ask for, try anything once.

BARITONE: Yeah. And what's relevant is telling the story of your time, it doesn't matter how you tell it. Just tell it.

SOPRANO: Yeah. Completely.

One of the most profound realizations that the cast of *BambinO* made was discovering how present the babies were during the performance and, more important, how that affected their delivery and confidence. Infants live in event time (see Chapter 1) or what Stern (2004) refers to by its Greek nomenclature, *Kairos*, meaning "the passing moment in which something happens as the time unfolds. It is a coming into being of a new state of things, and it happens in a moment of awareness. . . . It is a small window of becoming and opportunity" (p. 7). This ability to be in the present is crucial for infants. They are learning so much every day; the gift of immaturity allows for freedom from past baggage and future worries and for a generous amount of attention to the opportunities in the present. There were many opportunities in the opera experience, and as the musicians note, their own attention to moments of presence resulted in a meaningful exchange with the music and the audience.

This production provides an example of the tremendous potential for experiencing wonder when we can see life through the eyes of infants. It is a necessary component of creating change in the world: to disrupt the status quo, we need to ask "why?," and perhaps more important, oftentimes we need to ask "why not?" Capturing the essence of possibility is a reward for attending to children, who are free from the burdens of adult responsibility and the feeling of disenchantment that we experience when we've lost our vision of or hope for a safer, more caring society. We need to find the joy in mutual recognition in seeing and being seen by children to motivate our professional work: this is why we teach.

7

The Musical Legacies of Childhood and Children

> For we live with those retrievals from childhood that coalesce and echo throughout our lives, the way shattered pieces of glass in a kaleidoscope reappear in new forms and are songlike in their refrains and rhymes, making up a single monologue. We live permanently in the recurrence of our own stories, whatever story we tell.
> —Michael Ondaatje (2007, p. 135)

Reflecting on our childhood memories and our experiences with children help us retain, recapture, and reconsider the past and present experiences of music in our lives, and to make thoughtful, informed decisions regarding how to educate our students. Ondaatje, a Sri Lankan–born Canadian poet and novelist, uses the kaleidoscope to provoke an image of how the memories of our childhoods help us understand our current existence. The stories shared in this volume tell us that early experiences figure prominently in our musical memories and impact our adult lives. Moments of musical epiphany linger in our consciousness to secure our identity as musicians. We each have our own single monologue that changes with new encounters with music and with people, and with reiterations of our storied texts under multiple circumstances.

There are several themes that are woven through the chapters of this book. One recurring subject concerns the affordances that music provides for solitary introspection and social relatedness, turning the kaleidoscope from the within-person view, to see what is created between individuals in family, peer group, and ensemble settings. Another theme explores the ways in which our musical paths are influenced by dispositions, development, access, and participation, and how outcomes can be both predicted and surprising, welcomed and resisted. It is through the intersection of all these factors that we define our current selves and are defined by others.

The musical autobiographies of graduate students, and documented observations of children making music on their own, tell us about the varied ways in which music functions in everyday life; they also provide clues to how we learn music. Children's proclivities toward invention and imagination are not inhibitors of learning to be thrown away in the name of maturity; they are strengths to be nurtured and cultivated both in ourselves and our students.

In this final chapter, I look at the gifts of childhood and children as the foundation of our current musicality and reflect on how we were culturally inducted into our roles as musicians. I trace how music is experienced and music's role in our evolving sense of self and our relationships with others. I also address the musical paths that we make, and the stability and change that shape them. Lastly, I consider the pedagogical power of trust, wonder, and empathy as suggested by Cobb's (1977) concept of compassionate intelligence. First, I begin with the compelling nature of music itself, which calls us to join.

Becoming Music

What's important is not necessarily learning *how to play music* but rather, *how to become music*. Finding one's placement and role in the world called music, in other words, is not about making sound on instruments. It is, I believe, the key to understanding the essence of life (Parker, 2016, p. 176).

As was stated in the first chapter, we are musical beings. We benefit from children's unmasked and spontaneous responses to music and music making. How did this show itself in the autobiographical data presented? Two major themes are highlighted here: Being Present, which refers to an attuned consciousness to sound, and Embodiment, that is, the experience of implicit knowing through the body.

Being Present

The data I have presented suggest we don't just *play* music, we *live* music. Children teach us how to do this. As infants, their responses to our musical cues urge us to weave singing, chanting, dancing, and rocking with them into the fabric of our daily lives. Later, the spontaneous songs of childhood function as a way to express real-time emotion, regulate action, or narrate recent history. Living music is characterized as living with a certain consciousness of time defined by engagement—a keen awareness of the potential in the present moment.

We know children are fully present when making or listening to music—they are living in event time rather than clock time, aware of possibilities offered in the immediate context while simultaneously anticipating the ever-emanating future. When we sing to a toddler, they are with us, listening intently and projecting what will come next, responding with either delight in expectation realized or with surprise at expectation denied. Through these responses the child pulls us into the moment, and for a brief period we share event time, when our only concern is continuing the interaction. We intuitively hypothesize and act, changing our offering to be more interesting, relevant, or challenging for the child, seeking to engage them.

Such attunement is also seen in creative adults, in something researchers have called "discovery orientation" (Csikszentmihalyi & Getzels, 1988). By attending to the discernable characteristics of a phenomenon, we enter event time by allowing those characteristics to invite possibilities for change.[1] Immersing ourselves in the moment of inquiry, we are carried into a continued quest, guided by curiosity, agency, and the clear goals that result from focused attention.

For many musicians, such as Stephen Nachmanovitch (1990, 2019), being in the moment is closely associated with improvisation: "Making art . . . derives its patterns from everything around us, in an interdependent network. We learn to work as nature does, with the material of ourselves: our body, our mind, our companions, and the radical possibilities of the present moment" (2019, p. 4). Musicians Raymond MacDonald and Graeme Wilson (2020) acknowledge the music making of children as improvisational, highlighting the agency demonstrated in children's musical play as representative in the adult performer's making spontaneous choices concerning what to play next.

---

[1] Anna Craft (2015) describes the cognitive process as "possibility thinking" in her analyses of young children's learning.

Embodied Music

Associated with living in the present moment, which reflects a collapsing of past and future into "a simultaneity of now," is the embodiment of musical sound, a melding of our acting and thinking selves. Embodiment demonstrates implicit knowing, as shared memories of childhood, such as Nathan's experiences with Bazzini's "Dance of the Goblins" (see Chapter 4) remind us. When we become the music, we cannot separate our position as dancer from the dance—we experience what flow researchers have called the "merging of action and awareness" (Csikszentmihalyi & Csikszentmihalyi, 1988).

Embodiment has been a theme occurring throughout this book, in discussions of children's ways of being in the world and in our responses of amazement to discovering how children can physically express characteristics we as adults hear as musical cues. In many of the autobiographies there were stories of children embodying musicians—memories of getting a new guitar and instantly becoming a rock star, playing Donnie and Marie Osmond with the neighbors, or singing as Nancy Wilson at the Apollo. Our own musical childhoods were most likely filled with similar embodied experiences with the music and musicians of the day. Such experiences served to enculturate us more deeply into the practices of our varied social circles.

The experience of embodiment—this merging of action and awareness—is one that we feel internally. It is our joining with the sonic environment that creates the glorious feeling of unity of movement and sound. Although it does not require interaction with another person, it was most likely introduced to us by someone and it may be enhanced, or at least changed, when others are participating with us. In the following section, I discuss the social contexts of music making and how we experience the individual and collective vis-à-vis intersecting modes of engagement, intention, and positionality.

Alone and with Others: The Social Contexts of Musical Experience

In his discussion of extraordinary individuals, Howard Gardner (1997) argues for a model that involves relationships between the self, the domain of study, and other people. In the previous section we looked at experiences generated by the musical domain, specifically, at the ways in which we engage in *becoming* music—living in the moments of musical unfolding and deepening our relatedness through embodied synchronization with the sounds. The individual experience can be considered gratifying on a personal level, reminiscent of Piaget's "pleasure at being the cause." However, social contexts are crucial in shaping our musicality and the preferences and practices that define our musical lives. Below, I comment on reflections on the sense of belonging students reported having experienced in a variety of sound groups, and the role of mutuality, that is, seeing oneself in another, what I am calling kinship. Later, I also address the perceptions of private and public conditions under which children's music making happens and the roles adults play both in facilitating it and in shutting it down.

Sound Groups: Providing Kinship through Mutuality and a Sense of Belonging

Participants situated many of their musical memories in a group context— being in the company of specific people created specific music experiences. Family is our first sound group, and it offers a varied playlist that may include music from parents, grandparents, and siblings, as well as groups with whom we engage regularly as extensions of the nuclear family, such as fellow church members and neighbors. Using Bronfenbrenner's (1979) model of concentric circles of influence, we can envision the ecology of family music as a mesosystem of multiple interactions.

Even in the limited context of family music, the stories revealed distinct opportunities for engagement. Many autobiographers wrote about how music presented by their mother had a different function from that of music presented by their father. Supported by the parenting literature (e.g., Stern, 2010), fathers were often remembered as being more playful and mothers more soothing, though this was not universal. For example, Matt, whose mother was a music teacher and played the cello (his instrument of choice), shared, "My father in particular has a singing voice that I find soothing and comforting to this day."

Stories of grandparents were more common than expected and comprised varied styles of interaction. There were many examples of grandparents "making special" (Dissanayake, 2000), meaning that they engaged with their grandchildren in ways that were distinct, giving them a sense of belonging and making them feel loved and appreciated beyond the parent-child context. The strength of these intergenerational bonds even transcends death—recall Christian's search for and subsequent delight upon finding a recording of his grandfather's band (see Chapter 3).

Music with siblings advantages the shared imagination of children who also share a family history and culture. I value the chances I've had as an adult to play music with my brother, a drummer. Our shared past enriches the present moments of performance, even as we are creating new memories. A family sound group assumes belonging and provides a context for common experience; we can find similar qualities of kinship with peers in musical settings, from the playground, to the classroom, to the ensemble. A spontaneous sound group is created in a public park through an invitational call "Na na na na na, you ca-an't catch me!" attracting other children who recognize this music as their music. In Chapter 4 you read how Elizabeth wanted to play the violin after seeing Sarah Chang play, because Sarah looked like her. Gary experienced mutuality when he found an ensemble whose members also sought performance challenges with the same rigor as he had. Many of us found this in a variety of secondary school ensembles or in college—settings in which we experienced kinship, where we encountered people whose passion for making music was recognizable and shared.

Many students reported enjoying playing in smaller, chamber-sized ensembles. I have hypothesized that this is due to a human need for knowing that what we do matters, to be aware of our contribution to the greater whole. Our relatedness to the group is one way of perceiving our role in the ensemble: we may have a solo or we may add our voice to the chorus—we may stand out or fit in. Such positionality comes from the social affordances in music activity, which offer a broad range of participative possibilities.

Returning to the metaphor of the kaleidoscope, we can look and see how the same musical experience can look different depending on the interactions between the person and context. The bits of glass are arranged in myriad ways; with a simple turn, we can see interpretive variations on the experience of musical affordances. Rather than positioning ourselves in terms of group performance (fitting in and standing out), we may engage with music in terms of its situatedness, feeling inside or outside the music, embodied or detached. Turn the kaleidoscope again, and we may see how our experience is represented cognitively through our implicit knowledge, unnamed and felt in the body, and our explicit thinking—what we can identify through language and recall directly. Turn the kaleidoscope once more, and we can see how the glass pieces arrange around an intensity of response to the affordances, vis-à-vis passive and active engagement.

This rearrangement of the same pieces into various patterns of understanding exemplifies the complexity of musical experience. When we consider the music ensemble context, the intricacies of variation increase to include each participant's memories and experiences. One of the greatest and most rewarding challenges in music education is to create kaleidoscopic beauty in which the richness of our differences can be experienced as artistic kinship and engender feelings of belonging.

Public and Private Selves

Another way to consider social conditions for music making is the intention of the music maker. Is it meant to be shared or to be kept concealed? Most of us would probably respond: "It depends." If we were practicing a technically difficult passage, we would most likely want to do that in private. If we curate and prepare a concert program, we do so with expressive intention—it is designed for sharing. Music is intimate and it is galvanizing. Parents sing to their infants in a private conversation, soothing them with vocal production reserved for this purpose alone. The same parents might go to a rock concert and sing along with the lead guitarist at full volume, joining with thousands of other people in attendance. So yes, it depends.

Children's spontaneous singing provides insight into the private and public domains of music making (Bjørkvold, 1992; Marsh, 2008; Moorhead & Pond, 1941–1951/1978). When children play with other children, they often sing in short, repetitive, and very rhythmic chant-like phrases that have a limited pitch range and often use invented syllables (as demonstrated in the public park example introduced earlier). When children sing alone, the function is different; instead of communicating with others, the function is more self-directed, intended to comfort, reflect, and imagine. The quality of these spontaneous songs is strikingly different from the group setting. Here, the melodies had a greater range, were rhythmically amorphous, and had descriptive lyrics that often reflected what had happened that day or what was happening in the present moment. Many of these songs were composites of invented and learned song; a typical borrowed excerpt heard in the United States is "E I E I O" from "Old MacDonald's Farm." The collage-like effect of these composite songs is one of free reflective improvisation accentuated with brief interjections of familiar, culturally salient material. It is a blending of the private and the public.

In a recent discussion with my sister, she divulged that when she walked home from school alone at age eight or nine, she would sing, while keeping surveillance for anyone who might be in earshot. She was creating her own private space, which, as the second child in a family of five children, was a rare commodity. It reminded me of a line from a popular musical of that era, Rodgers and Hammerstein's *Cinderella*: "In my own little corner in my own little chair, I can be whatever I want to be." Children use music to imagine, and they often do so privately with no intention of sharing, especially with adults.

In the autobiographical data, there were indications of the need for privacy such as Heejung's use of music as a "secret gate to [her] own world" (see Chapter 4). She differentiates between her presented "outward image of brightness and innocence" and her "secret melancholy" that she wants to protect from exposure. In their book *Childhood Secrets*, Van Manen and Levering (1996) write about children's need for private places and solitary experiences to support their growth and development of an inner self. They note differences between privacy and secrecy. The former guarantees our control over our personal space and information and is valued for its protection from uninvited intervention and its provision of opportunities for self-reliance and autonomy. Channeling this independence, the latter provides an empowering sense of consequential action, promoting imaginative thought facilitated by the many possible interpretations of the secret object, place, or observed action.

Van Manen and Levering also point to the intimacy created when secrets are shared; it may be that music takes the form of a secret, and that sharing it with an audience or fellow performers creates an intimacy—intended or unintended. Jeremy revealed the discomfort he experienced singing at his mother's funeral: *"When I began to sing this song, everyone in the room disappeared and it was only me and her. I was singing my goodbyes to one of the only women I would ever truly love. Singing my woes to a room full of friends and family was one of the hardest things I ever had to do."*

Music making is a vulnerable yet compelling activity. By producing sound in a shared environment, we draw (often unwanted) attention to ourselves. I was waiting in a very large hall in New York City's Javits Center after receiving my COVID-19 vaccination. The typical wait time was fifteen minutes, so people were coming and going, seemingly detached from any group affiliation. During this pause in my day, I noticed a colorfully painted piano off to the side of the hall with a sign that read "Feel Free to Play." I was struck by the opportunity to do something personally satisfying and so casually walked up to this psychedelic upright piano that I could hide behind without being seen. It was a bit out of tune, but I didn't mind. I started to improvise, followed by a rendition of "What a Wonderful World," and ended with a cadenza and a sense of the aesthetic satisfaction I had sought out. My fifteen minutes were over, and I gathered up my things and headed toward the door. As I emerged from the piano, I suddenly heard applause from my fellow vaccinees, and felt surprised and a little embarrassed: for me it had been a private moment, albeit in a very public place. Watching children in the New York City subway, I have noted their ability to create their own spaces for music making, and how adult attention can halt the play and make the child feel ashamed for participating in musical play that was personally satisfying, yet with no visible practical function.

Our musical lives exist in a public forum, yet they bring private gratification. In sound groups we generally experience that gratification together, and this shared participation elevates our musical encounters. What can we learn about how to teach from acknowledging these interpersonal and intrapersonal connections with music? It is crucial to facilitate both a sense of self and a sense of belonging with others through planned activities that include personal exploration as well as ensemble playing and singing. Many autobiographies contained memories of feeling deeply connected to others when playing in ensembles and developed kinships based on those experiences. The social interactions that define our musical experiences and pathways are dependent on individuals' dispositions, development, and access to opportunities. In the following section, I trace the stability and changes that shape our childhoods and how, in turn, our childhoods shape our trajectories as musicians and teachers.

Making the Path: Interactions of Stability and Change over Time

It would be impossible to understand the Mahatma's stature and influence without knowing that he once was Moniya, and that the Moniya in him helped at strategic moments to free inner resources in himself and in his followers and to gauge, with a child's random sure-footedness, the actualities of the historical situation.

—Erikson (1969, p. 112)

This quote is from Erik Erikson's biography of Gandhi, which uses the Mahatma's own autobiography as source material. Moniya was his childhood name, and here, Erikson speaks to the legacy of childhood in adult life and to the significance of implicit knowledge he names "random sure-footedness." The habits and dispositions we accrue in our early years provide a vision of the self that remains with us, giving us stability to counter the unfamiliar physical and situational changes that define our existence.

My interpretations of musical memories have used family culture and dispositional traits to discuss stable enduring characteristics that first appear in childhood. Stability interacts with changes prompted by age-related development, the accessibility of social and material resources, and the ever-evolving present. In this section, I discuss the influence of our childhoods on the path-making decisions, the related outcomes, and the resilience and imagination required to become who we are and influence who we will be.

Stable Dispositional Traits and Dynamic Contexts of Music Making

McAdams (2015) writes that as social actors, we each come to the stage with a "unique presentational style" (p. 5). In its earliest form it is called temperament; with time, this style becomes identified as dispositions that carry on throughout the lifespan, contributing to a coherence of self. Dispositions reflect cultural values and have their roots in the legacy of our childhoods. The trait that addresses how we interact with others, Extraversion, is observable in the childhood dualities of public and private music making, as described above. The wide variety of behaviors considered as music participation suggest there are spaces for both Introverted and Extraverted activity in our musical lives and that we are not limited to a preset response to invitations to engage with music and musicians.

This notion of stability is not fixed—it is sensitive to the robustness of the environment; it is context-dependent. Family culture and individual dispositions are always operating, yet the intensity of influence can vary because it is moderated by the intentions inherent in the setting. For example,

Elise (see Chapter 4) surprised her parents by displaying an extroverted disposition when she was on stage performing with friends at school, as she was very introverted at home. Her presumed stable disposition was changeable—the new context allowed a reinvention of self as extroverted performer. The function of the stage as a space where one could "be whatever they wanted to be" has been a common theme throughout history, from Shakespeare to Stanislavski; the otherworldliness of the stage appeared in many participant stories. The transformative results of being on stage facilitated strong memories of Extraversion, as in this autobiographical account from internationally renowned musician Lang Lang regarding his first public performance experience at age five:

> I gave my first recital. In 1987, China still didn't know how to perform Western pieces; I was dressed in Peking Opera makeup, with a red face and heavy eye makeup. I looked like a little cat. I loved being on stage with the warm lights on me and the passionate applause from the audience. The stage felt like a sweet home to me. Right at that moment I decided to be a concert pianist. (2008, p. 35)

Being on stage was something many of us experienced, either in real life or in our imagination. The former setting was overwhelming for many of us because of the high stakes involved, while others, like Lang Lang, thrived in that environment. I am guessing that for him, it was a chance to be playful; his daily life was tightly controlled by his father, and on stage, he was able to be free and present the "fun-loving" aspect of his extraverted disposition. Those of us who spent more time on the imagined stage in our early years experienced extraversion through the imitation of musical models that encouraged imaginative thinking, or in one participant's words, "*Wait a second, what if I, Johnny, were one of these musical artists that I love so much?*" Musical play with friends and siblings was one of the most common themes found across a diverse spectrum of time and culture, including stories from Lebab in Harlem, United States (shared in 2016); from Lena in Athens, Greece (shared in 2004); and from Heejung in Korea (shared in 1999), who all talk about the role of the stage in their imaginative musical play. The R&B singer Patti LaBelle recalls her experience on the imaginary stage:

> Using a pencil for my Pall Mall [cigarette] and a rolled-up newspaper as my mike, I gave my first concert at age nine or ten. It was me, my mirror, and

my imagination. I played to a standing-room-only crowd. Honey, I killed them. That was the beginning, the start of my no-holds-barred concert performances. (1996, p. 43–44)

Another dispositional trait related to childhood play that has served musicians well in their path-making is Openness to Experience. Grammy Award–winning Beninese singer Angélique Kidjo reminisces about how her experience performing on stage not only required extraversion, but also an openness that brings with it the possibility to reinvent the presented self:

My mom always told me that you have to be spiritually naked when you walk onstage. You have to have a hell of an ego to go out there, but from the moment you do, your ego becomes secondary. Out there, you are in service of something bigger than you. Each time I'm onstage, I'm brand new. Anything can happen during a show. . . . The stage is a sacred place. (Kidjo, 2014, pp. 22–23)

Musicians who have a strong Openness disposition have an improvisatory spirit and can be uncomfortable with certainty. Libby Larson (in McCutchan, 1999) has expressed her maturation as a composer vis-à-vis a process of becoming comfortable with doubt, and she now feels distrustful of her work without it. Gandhi tapped into the "Moniya in him" to inform his path—he needed the child's "random sure-footedness," inferring a comfort with the unpredictability of the unknown.

There is an inherent trust in one's own actions in response to cues offered by the nature of the music itself, by performing partners and audience members, and by the physical environment. Trusting these cues outside of ourselves can lead to Bennett's (2001) notion of "pure presence" in which our implicit knowledge is brought forth and we experience attunement to music, others, and our surroundings.

Conscientiousness impacts the musical path by providing dispositional support for success. Neuroticism has the opposite effect, often blocking attunement with competing concerns. These two forces look different in everyone, mixing with Extraversion and Openness to create a relatively stable and unique amalgamation of dispositional traits. Stability and change are the forces that shape our growth and provide a coherent sense of self throughout the lifespan: stability is meaningful only in the context of change.

Kaleidoscopic Views of Developmental Change in Childhood

In viewing and interpreting our music experiences over the lifespan, we see how the path is made over time and how age-related changes influence our music making. We can also consider how music making might alter the projection of human growth and development (e.g., Habibi et al., 2018; Krause et al., 2014; Rauscher, Shaw, & Ky, 1993). We experience predictable biological and psychological changes that intersect with changes in living conditions as well as more stable cultural and dispositional factors—there are several kaleidoscopic turns we take. Next, I review the nature of developmental change and its relationship to musical experience, resourcing autobiographical works.

As infants we are predisposed for music making: we communicate through received and created vocalized patterns and respond to rhythmic rocking and speech—recall, for example. Kirstin's memories of being rocked and sung to as a young child (Chapter 3). The concomitant musical strengths in infancy are pitch matching and exploring the vocal range—a legacy that can be very enchanting as it invites adult interaction, which often takes the form of "motherese," a singsong, high-pitched way of speaking that often mimics the exaggerated pitch range. This caregiver-to-infant communicative style of interaction is encouraged by the baby's positive response.

I remember taking a walk with my then two-year-old niece, hearing a birdcall, and being amazed at her automatic response to the sound, matching the timbre and the pitch exactly. There is a palpable attunement in the way we begin our interactions with sound that is also present in the Openness disposition description, which includes words like creative, curious, and imaginative. Music may be an activity that provides a means to reinforce dispositional stability, fortifying a temperament by the affordances of meaningful action. Holding on to the ability to tune in to our surroundings is useful as we seek to belong in various musical groups, developing abilities to fit in and stand out. We are fully present and responsive to our environments.

Turning the kaleidoscope, we see how our musical life changes while leading into the period of early childhood, generally considered encompassing ages two or three through six or seven. Because we are more enculturated beings by this time, our musical behaviors are more recognizable to more people. Our sound group extends to include more demonstrable involvement with grandparents, siblings, and teachers and peers from preschool and kindergarten classrooms. Church was also a venue for significant experiences, especially for the Black community, as were extended families. Cognizant of all these resources, young children are not only social actors, but are becoming motivated agents, making choices about when, where, how, and with whom they engage in music making and furthering a sense of self fueled by the interactions with others.

The spontaneity of response and attunement beginning in infancy becomes a way of being in early childhood—it is when the qualities of Openness are at their most observable. Scientists, artists, and teachers often keep this childhood temperament as they maintain the curiosity and sense of wonder to find new questions to ask and problems to solve. Additionally, Extraversion usually surfaces in young children, expressed through their spontaneous singing and musical play practiced together. Music is a powerful organizer. It invites participation by rewarding the individual with great joy in the shared experience of mutuality.

Another turn, and we see changes as we enter later childhood: our sound groups become more differentiated; peers become more important, and we seek kinship with others who share a passion for the same music. We are more aware of the intersecting cultures of music in our lives and have developed specific ideas as to what constitutes music in our homes, at church, in our school classrooms, and on the playground. Each of these musical contexts calls for idiosyncratic skills and contributes to our overall sense of identity. Since it is also a time when we typically might start playing an instrument, taking lessons, and joining ensembles. We develop identities like "jazz trumpet player," "classical pianist," or "choir kid." Many autobiographers expressed strong relationships with their instruments that formed early, like Berkley, who wrote that his first time opening his trumpet case was like meeting a new friend for the first time (Chapter 4).

Turning again, we see our musical identities become more refined. During adolescence, our sound groups comprise people that like the music we like, reflecting both performance and listening preferences. We have accrued many ways of making meaning—we maintain the roles of social actor and motivated agent, retaining the abilities to focus on the present and project into the future. But we also begin to look at our past and become Autobiographical Authors, creating a coherent historical assessment of our path. We feel things deeply and are introspective, using music as an expressive strategy—reminiscent of the expressiveness experienced in our infancy before we had language (see Table 7.1).

Table 7.1 Developmental pathways of social action

Activation Relative to Life Period	Sound Group	Perspective (McAdams, 2015)	Meaning Making	Dispositional Sensitivity	Musical Strengths
Infancy	• Parent/Family	Social Actor	• Immense capacity for hearing and responding	Openness Extraversion	Vocal range Pitch matching Embodiment
Early Childhood	• and Extended Family • Preschool	and Motivated Agent	• Imagination • Capacity for wonder • Spontaneity • Discovery orientation		Learned Song Spontaneous Song Movement Experimentation
Middle Childhood	• and Peers		• Defined cultural idioms	Neuroticism Conscientiousness	Playing an Instrument (May start lessons)
Adolescent	• and Peer Groups	and Autobiographical Author	• Specificity of identity		
Adult	• New Roles		• Awareness of heritage • Coherence		

These developmental characterizations suggest possible directions the pathways may take as we walk them. Yet there are many other factors that interfere with the trajectories we plan. Unexpected disruptions, perceived failure, and insufficient resources can cause the paths to change, sometimes in dramatic ways.

Interruption, Trauma, and the Rerouting of Musical Lives

It is rare that our expectations for a musical life are realized in the ways we first conceive them. Unforeseen disruptions and opportunities appear, and we are forced to make decisions about how to proceed. The stories I read were defined by these junctures when change occurred suddenly or over time, and everything shifted. There were heart-wrenching experiences of traumatic loss of family members—some of the most difficult were shared by Jeremy in Chapter 5. Music assisted him in grieving, and ultimately in his recovery. Clara's loss of her teacher was devastating, and Claudia's traumatic health issues disrupted a probable career path as a performer. None of these disruptions was controllable by the musician-protagonist. Yet, these brave individuals were resilient, they persisted, and all were able to find renewal using music making and music teaching as intervention. After a year of mourning, Clara was able to return to playing her cello, motivated to realize the expectations of her deceased teacher. Jeremy acted with intention and agency, seeking renewal through performing in a choir. Claudia brought the same rigor and passion to her teaching that she had applied to her performance study. For many, the rewards of teaching music provided the emotional sustenance to withstand disruption.

Resistance, Renewal, and Resilience

Disruption can also be purposeful, in response to situations in which the quality of musical experience needs to be interrupted. Chamber music was a resource utilized by many autobiographers: examples include Elisa's renewal experienced when, after years of performing as a soloist, she began playing in a piano trio, and Ruth, whose favorite performance setting was a woodwind quintet and who talks about the excitement when her part—her contribution—is "exposed." The importance of being heard and the feeling of being in harmony with others are strong motivators for musical action, recalling the temporal experience of simultaneously fitting in and standing out.

We seek these opportunities for consequential action to resist scripts of insignificance and isolation. Music provides us a way to be together in which we retain our individual integrity. I have a strong memory of witnessing fleeting moments of synchronicity coming from the random chaos of nature. It was in Malaysia, and our guides were driving us in the dark of night far into the countryside. We stopped at a small café with a boating dock nestled over a small river. Our guides helped us onto the small vessels, and we followed the narrow waterway's twists and turns. Suddenly there appeared a few flashes of light—they were fireflies! This small ensemble grew into an orchestra of hundreds of lights flashing randomly, but if you waited long enough there would be a sudden unison flash bounded by complete darkness. This coming together of what seemed so sporadic felt miraculous, a visual metaphor for the coming together of sounds.

Disruption and renewal can reset our musical pathways and change our identities as musicians. Music teachers have much to do with the trajectories of students' musical lives—the power they have to confirm or deny our musical potential is salient in the autobiographical data. I found a particularly troubling example in a *New York Times* feature called "Metropolitan Diary" in which people reveal personal experiences that have potential to resonate with the readership. This entry written by Betty Baumel appeared on April 20, 2017, and is titled "Goodbye to the Listener's Row":

Dear Diary:
1937, second grade. The class is practicing a song to sing to our first-grade teacher, who is on maternity leave and coming to visit. I am really excited and singing my heart out. The teacher taps me on the shoulder and says, "Go sit in the listeners' row."

1941, the local settlement house. Private music lessons are 25 cents. My father would love to hear me play the violin. We go to Mr. Gerber's music store, and for $10 I get a violin, a bow, resin, and a cardboard carrying case. I have my first lesson and practice religiously for a week. The next week I return with quarter in hand and joyously play for my teacher. "Why don't you try another instrument?" he says.

1951, Brooklyn College. I am working toward my degree in elementary education. One of the required courses is how to teach music. At the end of the semester, the professor says, "Be sure you always have a record player to teach vocal music."

2017, the Riverdale Y senior center. Andy is returning to start a chorus. Everyone had so much fun with him last year. I work up my courage and go into the room. "Sure," he says, "come on and join us." After 80 years, I can sing.

Here, it seems the disposition for resilience miraculously overrides the experiences of rejection. Bonanno (2005) claims resiliency is more typical across populations suffering from trauma and adverse conditions than one might expect. However, neuroticism, especially the subsets insecurity and vulnerability, can be elevated in response to negative feedback, especially when delivered by a perceived expert.

In a multidisciplinary review, Ungar (2018) writes about seven characteristics of resilience that were common across systems of knowledge including published data from psychology, law, medicine, and additional subjects. They include general comments about how we define resilience through its relationship to adversity, and its process orientation. Ungar also cites qualities of a resilient system: it is open, dynamic, and complex; it promotes connectivity; it demonstrates experimentation and learning; and it includes diversity, redundancy, and participation. The autobiographers and scholars featured in this book have used these same descriptors to discuss musical experience. Could playing/singing together encourage and revive our capacity for resilience?

With this lens we recognize music's (and our own) openness and dynamism and are invited to experiment. Later, viewing the social emotional outcomes of musical engagement as belonging and mutuality, we can see how the power of a music education connects people with others and with themselves. In thinking about the role of educator in providing opportunities as a guide along the path, I briefly examine the idea of Teacher as Responsive Partner.

Teaching in Responsive Partnership

The Nobel laureate in literature Rabindranath Tagore wrote an autobiography titled *Boyhood Days*, first published in 1940. Reminiscences of his childhood reveal his motivation for creating a school in which students learned from the environment—from directly communing with their natural surroundings—and by engaging with the arts (Tagore, 1926/1997). He shunned his early teachers who considered instruction as a unidirectional delivery system and left traditional schooling because he wasn't encouraged to think for himself. It was his brother, Jyotidada, who became his first real teacher.

> I was twelve years his junior. It was amazing that I could attract his notice, despite this vast difference in age. More surprising still was the fact that he never silenced me by rebuking my precocity during our interchanges. Hence, I never lost the courage to give my thoughts free rein. (1940, p. 52)

Tagore describes a particular context in which the teacher's role of "responsive partner" calls upon the love of language and cultivates his poetic sensibility. He writes of when the family piano was delivered: "The fountain of my music now began to play. Running his fingers over the piano keys, Jyotidada composed rhythmic melodies in ever-new styles. He would keep me beside him. It was my task to provide an instant supply of words to accompany those racy tunes, holding the notes in place" (p. 52).

Tagore was sensitive to his significant contribution to the music making; he knew that his words would "hold the notes in place." This feeling of musical partnership that is experienced with a mentor is woven through most of the autobiographies presented. One of the most stunning examples is from Ruth's story in Chapter 5 in her description of playing with clarinetist Paquito D'Rivera in a master class: *"I can still feel the magic that surrounded my body as his notes surrounded mine like a glove, and he added an improvised harmonized part over mine."*

If music is a socially constructed activity, how can we as teachers engage in responsive musical partnership with our students? What does a responsive partnership look like across the lifespan? It starts in infancy. I remember quite vividly the astonishing clarity that I experienced at an international conference I attended many years ago. There were two different presentations on music making with babies. In the first the adult firmly grasps the legs of the baby and sings a song, moving the knees up toward their face to the pulse of "Row, row. row the boat. . . ." In the second presentation, the adult cupped the heel of the baby, attending to and gently supporting the baby's effort to move.

What constitutes support changes throughout human development. In the early childhood years, we support learning by honoring the musical possibilities in our environments, and by providing time in which to explore and imagine.

We also watch for invitations to respond to musical cues and are careful not to interrupt what may be private moments of creation. Later in middle childhood, we provide access to opportunities to try on various musical identities. Designing activities that are musically authentic and culturally meaningful supports these children's desires to play and sing sounds they recognize as music, and to see themselves as musicians. Leading into adolescence, students experience partnerships in traditional and non-traditional ensembles: following the teacher-conductor in a symphonic band, enjoying the responsivity of trading fours in a jazz quintet, and adding harmonies and solo passages in response to a garage band's improvisational excursion. We must be vigilant in our attention to these markers of childhood culture as they interact with family culture and disposition. In the final section I revisit Edith Cobb's conceptualization of Compassionate Intelligence and what it means for music education.

Empathy, Trust, and Wonder: A Pedagogy of/for Children

This realignment of the relation between the meaning of experience and culturally created information systems in terms of more contemporary knowledge is like the child's continued early experimentation with the links between perception and words during the process of creating [their] world image. And the process markedly resembles the method of the poet in creating the world of the poem. You need dynamic plastic fields of thought, language is an instrument of exploration, not a tool for the exposition of facts. (Cobb, 1977, pp. 108–109)

Throughout our lifespan we are striving to know ourselves through our interactions with others. We are also seeking to know the world through creating expressive representations of our experiences. This is what music offers: a chance to play with sounds, both literally and metaphorically figuring out who are in the world. The purpose of this book was to reacquaint us with the value in both children's artistic ways of being and our own autobiographic reflections on childhood. In doing this, we are reminded of our strengths and vulnerabilities, of the rewards we reap and the influence we impart in the social interactions of teaching and learning. Children experience and demonstrate familiarity with empathy, trust, and wonder—the key components to a compassionate intelligence.

Compassionate Intelligence: Exercising Empathetic Understanding

> If cultural attitudes could be shifted toward a recognition of human desire to exercise a compassionate intelligence, not only as tool and method but also as the chief human survival function, we would, I believe, find ourselves capitalizing on the human impulse to nurture, cultivate, and extend this vast potential. (Cobb, 1977, p. 111)

Cobb considers compassion as the "chief survival function" and calls out the medical and educational professions as "highly evolved forms of nurture" (p. 110). Some may argue with Cobb's premise, yet so much of what we truly care about is a motivated by a "human impulse to nurture, cultivate, and extend this vast potential" for compassion. The word "compassion" is defined as "sympathetic consciousness of others' distress together with a desire to alleviate it" (Merriam-Webster, n.d.). Music awakens our sense of kinship and through seeing ourselves in others who are known to us through musical collaboration. This is what I experienced in the Simunye concert in South Africa, when the Sdasa Chorale from Soweto joined with I Fagiolini from Oxford to create something new, reflective of their two distinctive styles.

Whether it be parent-child, teacher-student, peer-peer, or even performer-audience relationships—we are priming our accessibility to compassionate intelligence as we resonate in synchrony with others. Such encounters allow us to join our companions in sympathetic action to experience what they are feeling. Tuned in to musical expression and response, we strive to secure empathetic knowledge of another. Such focused action keeps compassion from becoming pity, which suggests a detached judgment of "otherness," rather than a "sympathetic consciousness of others." When we couple compassion with "intelligence" we ascribe value and "know-how" to the acts of alleviating distress and being good to others.

Relatedly, many students spoke of the strong emotional response to participating in music ensembles as something "greater than themselves." The potential for self-transcendence when engaging musically with others is key to understanding compassionate intelligence, as it is guided by a need to know how best to support and nurture music making. Reminiscent of flow experience, we can be optimally engaged and directed by compassionate intelligence, stepping outside our own concerns to offer our best selves to those we teach and those for whom and with whom we perform.

The transitions from full-time performing career to the teaching profession were marked by language that suggests the need for empathetic understanding. Remember Kokoe, who compared her experience performing with an ensemble at fourteen years of age to a teaching experience she had at age thirty. It is an example of how nurturing performance skills in her students resulted in an empathetic moment—a chance to see and feel with them something she had originally encountered earlier in her life: "It is incredible to have these experiences that live on in my memory and how I recall certain events that have shaped my life; and now how I am giving my students the opportunity and tools to experience unforgettable musical memories."

We are music teachers because we have firsthand knowledge of how it feels to be musical; we can empathize with student experiences, both the struggles and the triumphs. Below, I discuss the power of trust—a construct that has been uncomfortable for many mainstream music education scholars because it is equated with a loss of control. Looking at how children learn and grow, I make an argument for a pedagogy involving practices that honor the child's potential for and desire to "be good" and offer trustworthy authentic, collective musical experiences.

Expecting Goodness: Developing a Mindset of Trust

Compassionate intelligence permits the kind of understanding and sharing of "otherness" that we call "identification." To generalize this ability as a skill in learning would lead to the use of the humanities seldom encountered today.

When generalizing about the possibility of applying methods of identification and compassionate insight to the understanding of motivation ... we must recognize the destructiveness in ourselves as well as in others (which is essentially implied by the Socratic axiom, "Know thy self"). At the same time this knowledge needs to be matched by an awareness that at some time every human being experiences a profound longing to be good. This level of insight or truly compassionate intelligence requires an attitude of humility about knowledge as the first step. (Cobb, 1977, p. 7)

Cobb's use of the word "identification" is what I have been calling mutuality, the ability to see oneself in another. Mutuality brings about meaningful participation and encourages a level of trust that leads to a willingness to take risks. Her caution concerning the possibilities of destructiveness in both ourselves and in others protects from the dangers of "blind trust," suggesting that we enter the teaching-learning space with eyes (and minds wide open. This call for self-reflection, coupled with what Cobb calls "humility about knowledge," can create a mindset of trust in the transformative qualities of music experience and the capacity of children to attend, engage, and "be good."

We facilitate goodness in students by informed assessments of their needs. Two examples of what that looked like in the presented stories include the choice of instrument and the freedom to choose one's own repertoire—each of these reflecting trust in the learner and a fearless humility of knowledge. When students can take responsibility for their music making they are more invested and more responsive to our expectations of goodness. When teachers expect goodness, students are more likely to achieve.

One of the most courageous strategies of trust in a musical setting is found in the orchestra teaching of Dr. Tammy Yi (2018). While working on a doctorate in music education, she taught middle and high school orchestra in a suburb of New York City. The population of the school was demographically split between the wealthy and the working poor. Her ensembles were made up of students from both groups, and when she began teaching there it was clear that the financially privileged families could afford supplemental instruction for their children, which gave them an advantage in auditioned seating placement. To disrupt this socially unjust practice, Dr. Yi initiated a random seating arrangement, where the students would be placed in different positions within each section. This was a profound change, especially for the violins, where first chair was a coveted placement saved for only the most traditionally prepared student. This mixing and remixing of positions led to the whole orchestra improving and becoming an award-winning ensemble. Her trust in the power of relationship and social justice efforts is a marvelous example of compassionate intelligence.

Wonder and Discovery: Encouraging Lifelong Inquiry

If we put aside idealization of permanence or set goals and observe growth and learning in childhood as a period of gradual transcendence from level to level, out of biological nature into culturally created worlds, we become more conscious of the contributions, in the shape of values and even skills, which these earlier phases of personal history and biocultural development make to the fully adult personality. We then find ourselves in position of the connection between biological history, and cultural history, with individual childhood as the link in the series in time. (Cobb, 1977, p. 101)

The legacies of childhood and children are foundational and leave an imprint on our adult lives. We are enculturated into being from our biological beginnings and are shaped by our physical and social environments. The stories throughout this book provide examples of this—Claudia's playful interactions with her father, Jeremy's early experiences in church, and Ruth's memories of her mother performing mariachi—revealing the contexts that guided our curiosity and the accompanying drive to understand. To support that drive, we need to honor the childhood legacy of wonder, to cultivate an awareness of what we do not know and hypothesize possibilities of what could be.

Wonder involves problem finding, a term used by creativity researchers in the 1950s and 1960s and adopted by Csikszentmihalyi in the 1980s to describe how we sustain engagement by finding new achievable challenges in everyday activity. Sustained engagement is fueled by the need to explore, a quality of childhood behavior linked to learning (e.g., Piaget, 1962). As mentioned earlier in the book, his use of the term "discovery orientation" referred to a disposition for wonder, analogous to what McAdams calls Openness to Experience. We start with the awareness of something in our environment that causes us to wonder, challenging us to explore its potential, which leads to discovery. Discovery, therefore, is an outcome of wonder.

What might happen if we used wonder as a teaching strategy and introduced musical materials that were malleable and challenged students to inquire about possibilities: "What if . . ." or "let's try . . ."? Instead of a closed system emanating from an omniscient knowledge keeper, children can be encouraged to expand or extend or anticipate the given, playing with the conventional properties of space and time discussed in Chapter 1.[2] When children's proclivity for wonder and exploration are supported, their sense of inquiry is nurtured; they can receive the gift of discovery. Such gratification

---

[2] Expansion and Extension each require a change in space; however, Extension also suggests manipulations of time. Anticipation involves an attempt to compress time, to bring the future into the present (Custodero et al., 2002; Custodero, 2005).

is often robbed from them when education is only delivered via a didactic approach of "telling."

Several of the presented autobiographies contained memories that involved discovery. They were examples of intrapersonal realizations that resulted from informal settings. In telling the story of her early years, Lina discussed how she discovered the wholeness of music through spending time with her musical grandfather with whom she "learned how to listen to the music of nature and the music inside" of herself and that she "discovered and felt the wholeness of music." Claudia wrote about finding the sustain pedal on her piano in middle childhood and noted that "the discovery was overwhelming." Tanya reflected on her high school performance on the electric bass: "Within a millisecond of a change in the chord, I have discovered peace and perfection within the music, myself, and the entire world."

In each of these examples, the discovery reflects a sense of agency coupled with joy and gratitude. How can teachers nurture this childhood legacy of wonder, exploration, and discovery in ourselves and our students? It is a matter of both losing and finding oneself and the dance between living in the moment and constant reflection. It is an improvisation of life.

Epilogue: Childhoods in Flux: Considering Consequences of a Global Pandemic

Six years before COVID-19 became a global threat, Montuori (2014) exclaimed:

> Solid modernity, built on notions of order, stability, equilibrium, rationality, has given way to a "liquid" modernity, a Heraclitean world of constant change and disequilibrium. We are in a transitional moment, where one world is dying but a new one has not emerged. Uncertainty rules.

This change in the pacing of knowledge production and the notion of uncertainty came to a head when the WHO made their announcement in March 2020. Suddenly we were confronted with the results of being quarantined, masked, learning remotely, and losing people close to us. How have the legacies of children and childhoods been affected over the past years of global pandemic? How will the experiences of isolation, having faces covered and voices muffled, and relating to one another on screen shape the sensibilities of the children we teach? In social spaces, families, classmates, and friends have had their relationships disrupted by separation and fear. Intimacy is delivered at a distance, and the feelings of seeing others and being seen are modified. What have we lost? What, if anything, have we gained?

Music as a Social Tool

It was clear in the chapters that preceded that we saw music as a means of socialization. In our early years, it was with our families and as we got older it was our peers and teachers. During the pandemic, these units were redefined—families were limited to those living together; there were no extended family members like aunts or uncles or grandparents around to share the childcare duties or impart their wisdom. Although these losses were mostly temporary and children were often reunited with their loved ones, there were 529,000 deaths (Woolf, Chapman, and Lee, 2021) in the United

States alone that occurred during the first year of COVID-19. Given that these were mostly older adults, many children ended up missing out on the primal and permeating legacy of grandparents and the learning to be together that they taught.

They also missed out on the legacies that peers provided through kinship. Isolated from classmates and playmates, older children (in middle childhood) were often left alone to work through their learning issues rather than looking to their friends or joining performance groups to access ideas about identity and belonging. Adolescents were at a distinct disadvantage, as their daily interactions were mainly with parents, the very people from whom they were pulling back in efforts to be independent. Children of all ages spent most of their time with families—parent(s) and child(ren) were brought together in ways they had not experienced before.

Parents as Teachers: Finding Time and Spaces for Learning

One of those ways of being brought together was experiencing the family home as classroom. Families with preschool and primary school–aged children were burdened with the extra stress of managing increased responsibility for their education, as institutions usually carrying out that job were often closed or operating with minimal assistance. Taking on this role of teacher created a problem for many parents, especially mothers, who often had to give up their employment to attend to their children.

Tools necessary to bridge the gap between school and home were often computers. The teaching was online, and not all parents were prepared. There was a problem with digital literacy for many parents; many lacked basic access to computers and the internet. People of color were predominantly affected, as they were more likely to live in areas that were underresourced (Nichols, 2020). As a result of these problems, parents were often unequipped to carry their children through the COVID-19 crisis.

Our moments of interaction with children—the "pure presence" we shared with them previously—have changed. Consider the baby opera *BambinO*, where the infants and performers experienced "circles of wonderfulness." These one-on-one experiences, where adults were surprised and delighted by children's responses, are now less common—we may have temporarily lost the privilege of basking in moments of pleasure with one another and to see children as teachers in the hierarchy of control known as Zoom.

Scientists have found that time spent on screens by students has led to a depersonalization, a detachment of self from adults and the environment (Ciaunica et al., 2021). This detachment from the world was felt by most people, in varying degrees of significance: parents who have experienced trauma because of COVID-19 have passed this on intergenerationally, leading to a greater number of children whose mental health has suffered because adults are suffering. However, the adage "If Mama ain't happy ain't nobody happy" can also be turned around: parental resilience has also been linked to childhood well-being, and it appears that less-stressed parents mean less-stressed children (Marzilli et al., 2021).

Renewing Enchantment and Synchronicity

It seems important, then, to take care of ourselves, as our mental well-being determines that of our children. We can do this by seeking enchantment and synchronicity. According to Montuori (1989), to thrive during a time of uncertainty we need to develop creative, complex, and collaborative competencies that sustain us. In this final section I offer commentary on what the pandemic taught us and what we need to be aware of moving forward.

We were able to maintain creativity by turning our attention to production over performance. Screens became our palettes for imagination, where we could control parameters of sound and silence and we didn't need to worry about being in sync with others. We became producers of sound: composing and responding to the needs of the music itself, rather than directly with the people who made it. Although successful in engaging us in the final product as musical, this habit robs us of our in-the-moment definition of musical time and the spontaneous changes that are a result of our listening and playing together.

Production also allowed us to create interpretative complexities and autonomy within the limitations of the computer screen. Videotaped lessons became tools of agency where children could control what they watched, seeing more or less of a skill demonstration depending on what they feel they needed. This worked well for some, but it lacked the immediate give-and-take of a natural educational environment—the moments of connection and changes in direction that happen when music performance is experienced live.

The pandemic has challenged us in music education to turn the kaleidoscope in new directions. A few have been successful, but we must get more creative in joining together in synchronous performance, so that can we draw upon the enchantment that allows us to capitalize on the mutual experience of adults and children both in the music we make and the education we provide.

References

Abeles, H. (2009). Are musical instrument gender associations changing? *Journal of Research in Music Education, 57*(2), 127–139. https://doi.org/10.1177/0022429409335878

Abeles, H. F., & Porter, S. Y. (1978). The sex-stereotyping of musical instruments. *Journal of Research in Music Education, 26*(2), 65–75. https://doi.org/10.2307/3344880

Barkin, E. R. (1989, May). *"Music as a way of life"* [Paper presentation]. Taiwanese Composers' Forum, Taipei, Taiwan.

Barrett, M. S. (2010). Musical narratives: A study of a young child's identity work in and through music making. *Psychology of Music, 39*(4). https://doi-org.tc.idm.oclc.org/10.1177/0305735610373054

Bateson, P., & Martin, P. (2013). *Play, playfulness, creativity, and innovation*. Cambridge University Press.

Bennett, J. (2001). The enchantment of modern life: Attachments, crossings, and ethics. Princeton University Press.

Bjørkvold, J. R. (1992). *The muse within: creativity and communication, Song and Play from childhood through maturity*. MMB Music.

Blacking, J. (1995). *Music, culture, & experience: Selected papers of John Blacking*. University of Chicago Press.

Bonanno., G. A. (2005). Resilience in the face of potential trauma. *Current Directions in Psychological Science, 14*(3), 135–138.

Bornstein, M. H., & Tamis-LeMonda, C. S. (2014). Parent-infant interaction. In J. G. Bremner & T. D. Wachs (Eds.), *Wiley-Blackwell Handbook of Infant Development* (2nd ed., Vol. 1) (pp. 460–484). Wiley-Blackwell.

Bowlby, J. (1982). *Attachment*. Basic Books.

Bronfenbrenner, U. (1979). *The ecology of human development: Experiments by nature and design*. Harvard University Press.

Bronfenbrenner, U. (2001). The bioecological model of human development. In M. J. Smelser & P. B. Baltes (Eds.), *International Encyclopedia of the social and behavioral sciences* (pp. 6963–6970). Elsevier.

Buchanan, A., & Rotkirch, A. (2016). Introduction. In Buchanan, A. & Rotkirch, A. (Eds.), *Grandfathers: Global perspectives* (pp. 3–20). Palgrave Macmillan.

Calì, C. (2015). Music in family: Experiences of mutuality in middle childhood. (Doctoral Dissertation). (ProQuest, UMI Dissertations Publishing, 3707244).

Calì, C. (2020). Music in family dynamics and relationships: a case study. *Qualitative Research in Music Education, 2*(1), 63–89.

Campbell, P. S. (2010). *Songs in their heads: Music and its meaning in children's lives*. Oxford University Press.

The Chinese classics: Translated into English with preliminary essays and explanatory notes by James Legge. Vol. 2: The life and teachings of Mencius. 1875. N. Trübner.

Ciardi, J. (1959). *How does a poem mean?* The Riverside Press.

Ciaunica, A., McEllin, L., Kiverstein, J., Gallese, V., Hohwy, J., & Woźniak, M. (2022). Zoomed out: digital media use and depersonalization experiences during the COVID-19 lockdown. *Scientific Reports, 12*(1). https://doi.org/10.1038/S41598-022-0765-8.
Cirelli, L. K., Wan, S. J., & Trainor, L. J. (2014). Fourteen-month-old infants use interpersonal synchrony as a cue to direct helpfulness. *Philosophical Transactions of the Royal Society B, 369*: 20130400. http://dx.doi.org/10.1098/rstb.2013.0400
Clifton, T. (1983). *Music as heard: A study in applied phenomenology*. Yale University Press.
Cobb, E. (1977). *The ecology of imagination in childhood*. Teachers College Press.
Conrad, R. (1998). Darwin's baby and baby's Darwin: Mutual recognition of observational research. *Human Development, 41*(1), 47–64. https://doi.org/10.1159/000022568
Craft, A. (2015). Possibility thinking. In S. Robson & S.F. Quinn (Eds.), *The Routledge International Handbook of Young Children's Thinking and Understanding*, (pp. 416–432). London: Routledge.
Csikszentmihalyi, M. (1979). *Beyond boredom and anxiety*. Jossey-Bass.
Csikszentmihalyi, M. (1990). *Flow: The psychology of optimal experience*. Harper & Row.
Csikszentmihalyi, M. (1997). *Finding flow*. Basic Books.
Csikszentmihalyi, M., & Csikszentmihalyi, I. (Eds.) 1988. *Optimal experience*. Cambridge University Press.
Csikszentmihalyi, M., & Getzels, J. W. (1988). Creativity and problem finding in art. In F. H. Farley & R. W. Neperud (Eds.), *The foundations of aesthetics, art, & art education* (pp. 91–116). Praeger Publishers.
Csikszentmihalyi, M., & Rathunde, K. (1993). The measurement of flow in everyday life: Toward a theory of emergent motivation. In J. E. Jacobs (Ed.), *Current theory and research in motivation, Vol. 40. Nebraska Symposium on Motivation, 1992: Developmental perspectives on motivation* (pp. 57–97). University of Nebraska Press.
Custodero, L. A. (2005). Being with: The resonant legacy of childhood's creative aesthetic. *Journal of Aesthetic Education, 39*(2), 36–57. https://doi:10.1353/jae.2005.0015
Custodero, L. A. (2006). Singing practices in ten families with young children. *Journal of Research in Music Education, 54*, 37–56. https://doi:10.2307/3653454
Custodero, L. A. (2008). Musical portraits, musical pathways: Stories of meaning making in the lives of six families. In J. Kerchner & C. Abril (Eds.), *Music learning and teaching throughout our lives* (pp. 79–92). Rowman and Littlefield.
Custodero, L. A. (2009). Intimacy and reciprocity in improvisatory musical performance: Pedagogical lessons from adult artists and young children. In S. Malloch & C. Trevarthen (Eds.), *Communicative musicality: Exploring the basis of human companionship* (pp. 513–530). Oxford University Press.
Custodero, L. A., Britto, P. R., & Xin, T. (2002). From Mozart to Motown, lullabies to love songs: A preliminary report on the Parents Use of Music with Infants Survey. *Journal of Zero-to-Three, 23*(1), 41–46.
Custodero, L. A., Calì, C., & Diaz-Donoso, A. (2016). Music as transitional object and practice: Children's spontaneous musical behaviors in the subway. *Research Studies in Music Education, 38*(1), 55–74. https://doi.org/10.1177/1321103X15612248
Custodero, L. A., Chen, J. J., Lin, Y. C., & Lee, K. (2006). One day in Taipei: In touch with children's spontaneous music making. *Proceedings of the International Society for Music Education Early Childhood Commission Seminar, "Touched by Discovery,"* 84–91.
Custodero, L. A., & Johnson-Green, E. A. (2003). Passing the cultural torch: Musical experience and musical parenting of infants. *Journal of Research in Music Education, 51*(2), 102–114. https://doi.org/10.2307/3345844

Custodero, L. A., & Johnson-Green, E. A. (2008). Caregiving in counterpoint: Reciprocal influences in the musical parenting of younger and older infants. *Early Child Development and Care, 178*(1), 15–39. https:// doi.org/10.1080/03004430600601115

Damasio, A. (1999). *The feeling of what happens: Body and emotion in the making of consciousness*. Harcourt Brace.

Damasio, A. R. (2010). *Self comes to mind: Constructing the conscious brain*. Pantheon Books.

Darian-Smith, K., & Pascoe, C. (2013). Children, childhood, and cultural heritage: Mapping the field. In K. Darian-Smith & C. Pascoe (Eds.), *Children, childhood, and cultural heritage* (pp. 1–17). Routledge.

Deci, E. L., & Flaste, R. (1996). *Why we do what we do*. New York: Penguin.

DeLorenzo, L. C. (2012). Missing faces from the orchestra: An issue of social justice? *Music Educators Journal, 98*(4), 39–46. https://doi.org/10.1177/0027432112443263

DeNora, T. (2000). *Music in everyday life*. Cambridge University Press.

Dissanayake, E. (1995). *Homo aestheticus: Where art comes from and why*. University of Washington Press.

Dissanayake, E. (2000). *Art and intimacy: How the arts began*. University of Washington Press.

Dissanayake, E. (2013). Genesis and development of "Making Special": Is the concept relevant to aesthetic philosophy? *Rivista Di Estetica*, (54), 83–98. https://doi.org/10.4000/ESTETICA.1437

Elkind, D. (2007). *The power of play: How spontaneous, imaginative activities lead to happier, healthier children*. Da Capo Lifelong Books.

Erikson, E. H. (1969). *Gandhi's truth: On the origins of militant nonviolence*. New York: W. W. Norton.

Ferneyhough, C. (2012). *Pieces of light: The new science of memory*. Profile Books.

Field, T. (2010). Postpartum depression effects on early interactions, parenting, and safety practices: A review. *Infant Behavior and Development, 33*(1), 1–6. https://doi.org/10.1016/j.infbeh.2009.10.005

Fisher, P. (1998). *Wonder, the rainbow, and the aesthetics of rare experiences*. Harvard University Press.

Frith, S. (1996). Music and identity. In S. Hall & P. du Gay (Eds.), *Questions of cultural identity*, (pp. 108–128).

Gabrielsson, A. (2011). *Strong experiences with music: Music is much more than just music* (R. Bradbury, Trans.). Oxford University Press.

Gardner, H. (1997). *Extraordinary minds*. New York: Basic Books.

Gebesmair, A., & Smudits, A. (2001). *Global repertoires*. Routledge.

Gibson, J. J. (1977). *The theory of affordances*. Erlbaum.

Gluschankof, C. (2002). The local musical style of kindergarten children: A description and analysis of its natural variables. *Music Education Research, 4*(1), 37–49. https://doi.org/10.1080/14613800220119769

Goldberg, L. R. (1981). Language and individual differences: The search for universals in personality lexicons. In L. Wheeler (Ed.), *Review of personality and social psychology, 1* (pp. 141–165). Sage.

Gulbrandsen, L. M. (2012). Being a child, coming of age: Exploring processes of growing up. In M. Hedegaard, K. Aronsson, C. Højholt, & O. S. Ulvik (Eds.), *Children, childhood, and everyday life: Children's perspectives* (pp. 3–36). Information Age Publishing.

Habibi, A., Damasio, A., Ilari, B., Veiga, R., Joshi, A. A., Leahy, R. M., Haldar, J. P., Varadarajan, D., Bhushan, C., & Damasio, H. (2018). Childhood music training induces change in micro and macroscopic brain structure: results from a longitudinal study. *Cerebral Cortex, 28* (12), 4336–4347. https://doi.org/10.1093/cercor/bhx286

Hallam, S. (2010). The power of music: Its impact on the intellectual, social and personal development of children and young people. *International Journal of Music Education, 28*(3), 269–289. https://doi.org/10.1177/0255761410370658

Ilari, B. (2005). On musical parenting of young children: Musical beliefs and behaviors of mothers and infants. *Early Childhood Development and Care,* 175(7–8), 647–660. https://doi.org/10.1080/0300443042000302573

Ilari, B. (2018). Musical parenting and music education: Integrating research and practice. *Update: Applications of Research in Music Education, 36*(2), 45–52. https://doi.org/10.1177/8755123317717053

Johnson, M. (2015). *The meaning of the body: Aesthetics of human understanding.* University of Chicago Press.

Kemp, A. E. (1996). *The musical temperament: Psychology and personality of musicians.* Oxford University Press.

Kidjo, A. (2014). *Spirit rising: My life, my music.* New York: Harpers Collins Publishers.

Krause, N., Homickel, J., Strait, D. L., Slater, J., & Thompson, E. (2014). Engagement in community music classes sparks neuroplasticity and language development tin children. *Frontiers in Psychology.* https://doi.org/10.3389/fpsyg.2014.01403

Koops, L. H. (2014). Songs from the car seat: Exploring the early childhood music-making place of the family vehicle. *Journal of Research in Music Education, 62*(1), 52–65. https://doi.org/10.1177/0022429413520007

Koops, L. H. (2019). *Parenting musically.* Oxford University Press.

Lawler, S. (2000). *Mothering the self: Mothers, daughters, subjects.* Routledge.

Lesiuk, T. (2019). Personality and music major. *Psychology of Music, 47*(3), 309–324. https://doi.org/10.1177/0305735618761802

Levine, R. V. (1998). *A geography of time: The temporal misadventures of a social psychologist.* Basic Books.

Lum, C., & Whiteman, P. (2012). Children and childhoods. In C. Lum and P. Whiteman (Eds.), *Musical childhoods of Asia and the* Pacific (pp. 1–9). Information Age Publishing.

Malloch, S., & Trevarthen, C. (2009). *Communicative musicality: Exploring the basis of human companionship.* Oxford University Press.

Marsh, K. (2008). *The musical playground: Global tradition and change in children's songs and games.* University Press.

MacDonald, R. A. R., & Wilson, G. B. (2020). *The art of becoming: How group improvisation works.* Oxford University Press.

Marzilli, E., Cerniglia, L., Tambelli, R., Tromboni, E., DePascalis, L., Babore, A., Trtumello, C., Cimino, S. (2021). The COVID-19 pandemic and its impact on families' mental health: the role played by parenting stress, parents' past trauma, and resilience. *International Journal of Environmental Research and Public Health, 18* 11450. https://doi.org/10.3390/ijerph182111450.

McAdams, D. (2015). *The art and science of personality development.* Guilford Press.

McCutchan, A. (1999). *The muse that sings: Composers speak about the creative process.* Oxford University Press.

Mikulincer, M., Shaver, P. R., & Pereg, D. (2003). Attachment theory and affect regulation: The dynamics, development, and cognitive consequences of attachment-related strategies. *Motivation and Emotion, 27*, 77–102. https://doi.org/10.1023/A:1024515519160.

Miralis, Y. (2004). Manos Hadjidakis: The story of an anarchic youth and a "Magnus Eroticus." *Philosophy of Music Education Review, 12*(1), 43–54. https:// doi.org/10.1353/pme.2004.0007

Moorhead, G., & Pond, D. (1978). Music of young children. Santa Barbara, CA: Pillsbury Foundation for the Advancement of Music Education. Original work published in 1941.

Montuori, A. (1989). *Evolutionary competence: Creating the future. CIIS Faculty Publications.* 21.

Montuori, A. (2014). Un choc des mentalités: Incertitude, crŽativitŽ et complexitŽ entemps de crise. (A clash of mentalities. Uncertainty, creativity and complexity in a timof crisis. *Communications.* 95(2), 179-198.

Nachmanovitch, S. (1990). *Free play: Improvisation in life and art.* Penguin.

Nachmanovitch, S. (2019). *The art of is: Improvising as a way of life.* Novato, CA: New World Library.

Neumann, A. (2009). *Professing to learn creating tenured lives and careers in the American research university.* Johns Hopkins University Press.

Nichols, B. E. Equity in music education: access to learning during the pandemic znd beyond. *Music Educator's Journal,* 107(1) 68-70. http://doi.org/10.1177/00274321209451561

O'Donnell, J. (2013). *Les Paul: The lost interviews: Five never-before-published talks with a guitar genius.* CreateSpace Independent Publishing Platform.

Ondaatje, M. (2007). *Divisadero.* New York: Knopf.

Papousek, M. (1996). Musicality in infancy research: Biological and cultural origins of early musicality. In I. Deliege & J. A. Sloboda (Eds.), *Musical beginnings: Origins and development of musical competence* (pp. 37–55). Oxford University Press.

Parker, W. (2016). Becoming music: Building castles with sound. In A. Heble & M. Lave (Eds.), *Improvisation and Music Education: Beyond the Classroom*, (pp. 176–180). New York: Routledge.

Piaget, J. (1962). *Play, dreams, and imitation in childhood.* New York: W. W. Norton.

Pigrum, D. (2009). *Teaching creativity: "Multi-mode" transitional practices.* Continuum.

Pilkauskas, N., & Martinson, M. (2014). Three-generation family households in early childhood: Comparisons between the United States, the United Kingdom, and Australia. *Demographic Research,* 30, 1639–1652. https://doi.org/10.4054/DemRes.2014.30.60

Randall, W. L. (2015). *The narrative complexity of ordinary life: Tales from the coffee shop.* Oxford University Press.

Rasmussen, A. S., & Berntsen, D. (2009). Emotional valence and the functions of autobiographical memories: Positive and negative memories serve different functions. *Memory & Cognition,* 37(4), 477–492. https://doi.org/10.3758/MC.37.4.477

Rauscher, F. H., Shaw, G. L., & Ky, K. N. (1993) Music and spatial task performance. *Nature,* 365(6447), 611. https://doi.org/10.1038/365611a0

Roopnarine, J. L. (2015). *Fathers across cultures: The importance, roles, and diverse practices of dads.* Praeger.

Russ, S. W. (2013). *Pretend play in childhood: Foundation for adult creativity.* American Psychological Association.

Shafer, R. M. (1994). *The soundscape: Our sonic environment and the tuning of the world.* Destiny Books.

Siegel, D. J. (1999). *The developing mind: Toward a neurobiology of interpersonal experience*. Guilford Press.
Singer, D. G., & Singer, J. L. (1990). *House of make believe: Children's play and developing imagination*. Harvard University Press.
Sole, M. (2016). Crib song: Insights into functions of toddlers' private spontaneous singing. *Psychology of Music*, 45(2), 172–192. https://doi.org/10.1177/0305735616650746
Stern, D. N. (1985). *The interpersonal world of the infant: A view from psychoanalysis and developmental psychology*. Basic Books.
Stern, D. N. (2004). *The present moment: In psychotherapy and everyday life*. W. W. Norton.
Stern, D. N. (2010). *Forms of vitality: Exploring dynamic experience in psychology, the arts, psychotherapy, and development*. Oxford University Press.
Tagore, R. (1926/1997). A poet's school. In K. Dutta & A. Robinson (Eds.), *Rabindranath Tagore: an anthology* (pp. 248–261). London: Macmillan.
Tagore, R. (1940/2011). *Boyhood Days*. London: Hesperus.
Theodorakis, M. (2007). *Universal Harmony*. (M. Solman, Trans.). In G. Kugiumutzakis (Ed.), *Universal harmony, music and science in honor of Mikis Theodorakis* (pp. 75–102). Crete University Press.
Trehub, S. E. (2001). Musical predispositions in infancy. *Annals of the New York Academy of Sciences*, 930(1), 1–16. https://doi.org/10.1111/j.1749-6632.2001.tb05721.x
Trehub, S. E. (2003). Musical predispositions in infancy: An update. In I. Peretz & R. Zatorre (Eds.), *The cognitive neuroscience of music* (pp. 3–20). Oxford University Press. https://doi.org/10.1093/acprof:oso/9780198525202.003.0001
Trehub, S. E. (2009). Music lessons from infants. In S. Hallam, I. Cross, & M. Thaut (Eds.), *The Oxford handbook of music psychology* (pp. 229–234). Oxford University Press.
Trehub, S. E., Unyk, A. M., Kamenetsky, S. B., Hill, D. S., Trainor, L. J., Henderson, J. L., & Saraza, M. (1997). Mothers' and fathers' singing to infants. *Developmental Psychology*, 33(3), 500–507. https://doi.org/10.1037/0012-1649.33.3.500
Trevarthen, C., & Malloch, S. (2002). Musicality and music before three: Human vitality and invention shared with pride. *Zero to Three*, 23(1), 10–18.
Trevarthen, C. & Malloch, S. (2016). Grace in moving and joy in sharing: The intrinsic beauty of communicative musicality from birth. In S. Bunn, (Ed.), *Anthropology and beauty: From aesthetics to creativity*. Routledge.
Tudge, R. H., Mokrova, I., Hatfield, B. E., & Karnik, R. B. 2009. Uses and misuses of Bronfenbrenner's bioecological theory of human development. *Journal of Family Theory and Review*, 1, 198–210. https://doi.org/10.1111/j.1756-2589.2009.00026.x
Turino, T. (2008). *Music as social life: The politics of participation*. University of Chicago Press.
Turner, V. (1969). *The ritual process: Structure and anti-structure*. Aldine Publishing.
Ungar, M. (2018). Systemic Resilience: principles and processes for a science of change in contexts of adversity. *Ecology and Society* 23(4), 34.
Van Manen, M., & Levering, B. (1996). *Childhood's secrets: Intimacy, privacy, and the self reconsidered*. Teachers College Press.
Wallin, N. L., Merker, B., & Brown, S. (Eds) (2000). *The origins of music*. Cambridge, MA: The MIT Press.
Wiggins, J. (2011). Vulnerability and agency in being and becoming a musician. *Music Education Research*, 13(4), 355–367. https://doi.org/10.1080/14613808.2011.632153.

REFERENCES   165

Willox-Blau, P. (1990). Toward cultural integration: The career development of black musicians and the symphony orchestra. *Journal of Arts Management and Law, 20*(1), 17–36.

Winnecott, D. W. (1971). *Playing and reality.* Routledge.

Wittgenstein, L. (1968). *Philosophical investigations* (3rd ed., G. E. M. Anscombe, Trans.). Oxford: Basil Blackwell.

Woolf, S. H., Chapman, D. A., & Lee, J. H. (2021). COVID-19 as the leading cause of death in the United States. *Journal of the American Medical Association, 325*(2): 123–124. doi: 10.1001/jama.2020.24865.

Yi, Tammy S. (2018). Back of the orchestra: High school students' experiences with alternative seating practices. Doctoral dissertation, Teachers College, Columbia University. https://doi.org/10.7916/D8D80TW3.

Zatorre, R., Chen, J. & Penhune, V. (2007). When the brain plays music: Auditory-motor interactions in music perception and production. *National Review of Neuroscience, 8,* 547–558. https://doi.org/10.1038/nrn2152

Zur, S. S. (2007). *Cultural perspectives of experienced time: An investigation of children's music making as manifested in schools and communities in three countries* [Doctoral dissertation, Teachers College, Columbia University]. ProQuest Dissertations & Theses Global. https://tc.idm.oclc.org/login?url=https://www-proquest-com.tc.idm.oclc.org/dissertations-theses/cultural-perspectives-experienced-time/docview/304862556/se-2

Index

For the benefit of digital users, indexed terms that span two pages (e.g., 52–53) may, on occasion, appear on only one of those pages.

Tables and figures are indicated by *t* and *f* following the page number

"Adagio in g minor" (Albinoni), 74
Adelante Winds, 103
affect attunement, 57
"Alberti Bass," 3
Albinoni, Tomaso, 74
Allen, Peter, 19
Anderson, Marian, 79
autobiographical memory, 22

Baez, Joan, 64–65
ballet folklorico, 99–100
BambinO, 117–27, 119f, 156–57
Barkin, Elaine, 29
Baumel, Betty, 145–46
Baxani, Nita, 118
Bazzini, Antonio, 65, 70–71, 132
becoming music, 130, 132–33
Beethoven, Ludwig van, 13, 104
being present, 130–32
Bennet, 140
Bennett, 116–17
Berlin, Irving, 52
Bernstein, Leonard, 112–13
Berntsen, D., 22, 23, 24
Blacking, J., 10
Black performers, in classical music and opera, 79
Blodgett, Pat, 82–83
Bonanno, 146
Boyhood Days (Tagore), 146–47
Boyz2Men, 97
Brahms, Johannes, 74, 101–2
Brewer, Teresa, 44
Bronfenbrenner, U., 25, 27, 42, 133
Brown, James, 53–54

Calì, C., 114
call-and-response, 12–13
Canon in D, 109
Chang, Sarah, 79–80, 134
"Cheek to Cheek," 52
Childhood Secrets (Van Manen and Levering), 136
Ciardi, John, 2n.1, 6, 7
Cinderella, 136
"Cleanup Song," 12
Clifton, Thomas, 65
Clinton, Bill, 24
Cobb, Edith, 17–18, 24–25, 30–33, 31*t*, 111, 117, 125, 130, 148–53
coherence, continuity and, 27–28
comfort, music as, 12–14
communicative musicality, 44–45, 83, 114
compassionate intelligence, 32, 125, 130, 147–48, 150, 151
  empathetic understanding and, 149–50
  enchantment and, 116–17
Conrad, R., 114–15, 116
COVID-19 pandemic, 155–58
Crests, the, 69–70
Csikszentmihalyi, M., 85, 152
Custodero, Lori A., 31*t*

Damasio, Antonio, 10, 24, 55, 61–62, 63
"Dance of the Goblins," 65, 70–71, 132
"Dance of the Sugarplum Fairy, The," 9
"Dance with my Father Again," 96–97
dancing, 6–7, 8, 132
Darwin, Charles, 114–15, 116
"De Colores," 99
Denver, John, 19

developmental change in childhood, kaleidoscopic views of, 141–44, 143*t*
Diabelli, Anton, 104–5
discovery orientation, 27–28, 85, 131, 152
dispositions, 27–28, 141–42
   embodiment and, 65–67
   implicit knowing and, 62–67
   musical identity and, 84–85
   personality traits, motivating conditions and, 67–75
   for resilience, 146
   stable traits, dynamic contexts of music making and, 138–40
disruptions and renewals, in career trajectories of musicians, 87–107, 144–48
Dissanayake, E., 2, 57
Donny and Marie Osmond, 51–52, 132
"Don't Get Around Much Anymore," 42–43
D'Rivera, Paquito, 102–3, 109, 147
Dvořák, Antonín, 51, 82

Ebenezer Baptist Church, 89–90
ecologies, of childhood musical experiences, 24–26, 26*f*, 27, 38–40, 55–56
Ecology of Imagination in Childhood, The (Cobb), 17, 24–25
"Eine kleine Nachtmusik," 81
Ellington, Duke, 68
embodiment, 65–67, 114–15, 130, 132
emotion, 22–23, 24–25, 44, 55, 72–75, 140. *See also* feeling, of music
empathetic understanding, 149–50
empathy, trust, and wonder, in pedagogy for children, 148–53
enchantment, 116–17, 125–27, 157–58
encounters with children, legacy of, 111–13
enculturation, 53–54, 57–58, 132, 141–42, 152
Erikson, Erik, 137–38

family, as sound group, 38–43
family member roles, music and, 43–52, 55–56
feeling, of music, 8, 9–14

Ferneyhough, Charles, 23–24
Fisher, Phillip, 116
folk music, 53, 55–56, 99–100
"Forza del Destino, La," 74
fundamentalist perspective, in music education, 95–96
"Für Elise," 104

Gabrielsson, Alf, 23
Gandhi, 137–38, 140
Garcia, Jerry, 47–48, 58
Gardner, Howard, 132–33
generativity, teaching narratives and, 107–10
Getzels, J. W., 85
Glass, Philip, 6
Gluschankof, Claudia, 2
Goals 2000: The American Education Act, 24
"God Bless America," 3–4
"Goodbye to the Listener's Row" (Baumel), 145–46
goodness, expectation of, 150–51
grandparents, in childhood musical experiences, 48–50, 133–34
Grateful Dead, 47–48, 57

"Habanera," 64
Hadjidakis, Manos, 2
Hairspray medley, 71–72
"Haitian Fight Song," 68
"Happy Go Lucky Local," 68
"Happy to Be Stuck with You," 42–43
Hargreaves, David, 78–79
harmony, 6
Haydn, Franz Joseph, 6
Henderson, Skitch, 95
"His Eyes Are on the Sparrow," 96–97
historical self, childhood and, 18–21
Huey Lewis and the News, 42–43
Humes, Scot, 101

I Fagiolini, 57–58, 149
I Hate Music! A Cycle of 5 Kid's Songs for Soprano and Piano (Bernstein), 112–13
"I Know Who Holds Tomorrow," 42

INDEX

Imani Winds Chamber Music Festival, 102–3
"I'm a Person Too," 112–13
implicit knowing, 62–67, 130, 140
implicit musicality, 63–65
improvisation, 131, 135–36
infants, 114–15, 117–27, 141, 156–57
influence, patterns of, 27
instrument choice, 75–78, 84, 99–100, 151

Jesus, 111, 111n.2
"Jingle Bell Rock," 94
Johnson, Mead, 53–54

Kairos, 126
kaleidoscopic design, 30–33, 129–30, 134–35, 141–44
Kidjo, Angélique, 140
King, Martin Luther, Jr., 89–90
King Sanders, Nancy, 102
Koops, L. H., 42

LaBelle, Patti, 139–40
Lang Lang, 138–39
Lao Tzu, 111
Larson, Libby, 140
Lawler, S., 45–46
"Let It Be," 107–8
Levering, B., 136
Levine, R. V, 5

MacDonald, Raymond, 131
Magic Flute, The, 119–20
Makeba, Miriam, 64–65
Marsh, Kathryn, 2
Martinson, M., 48
Matthews, Dave, 66
McAdams, Dan, 30–32, 31*t*, 33, 61–62, 67–68, 69, 71, 74, 84–85, 107, 138, 152
McDermott, Phelim, 120–21, 124, 126
Mead, Margaret, 17
melody, harmony and, 6
memory
　accessing and sharing, 35–38
　autobiographical, 22
　childhood, 21, 62, 111, 129
　emotion and, 22–23, 24–25, 44
　in musical ecology, 24–25, 27
　of musical experiences, in autobiographies, 27–28, 35–38
　in musical identity, 27, 129
　truth, values and, 23–24
method, as mosaic, 17
Metropolitan Opera, 118, 119*f*
Mingus, Charles, 68
Montuori, 155, 157
motherese, 141
motivated agents, 61–62, 66, 67, 70, 141–42
Mozart, Wolfgang Amadeus, 97–98, 101–2, 119–20
Mozart Effect, the, 53–54
Murata, Setsuko, 103–4, 106
music
　becoming, 130, 132–33
　as social tool, 155–56
musical communication and communicative musicality, 11–13, 44–45, 83, 114
musical experience
　collective, 81, 150
　ecologies of, 24–26, 26*f*, 27, 38–40, 55–56
　grandparents in, 48–50, 133–34
　meaning of, 2–4
　memory of, 27–28, 35–38
　of movement, 5–8
　in music education for children, 15–16
　parents in, 43–48, 52, 57
　public-private duality of, 14
　siblings in, 50–52, 134
　social contexts of, 132–37
　of time, 4–5
musical expression, feeling of music and, 9–10
musical heritage, 58–59
musical identity, 28, 62–63, 65, 67, 83–85, 142
　dispositional traits and, 84–85
　instrument choice and, 75–78, 84
　memory in, 27, 129
　positionality in formation of, 83–84
　sound groups and, 142
musical kinship, 78–83, 133–35
musical legacy, 1–2
musical legacy, childhood and, 1–2

musical movement, 5–8, 10
musical play, 11–12, 50–52, 83, 111–12, 131, 136–37, 139, 142
musical selves, 55–59, 61–62, 83–84, 135–37
musical time, 4–5
music autobiographies, 18–20
   assignment, 20*t*
   on chamber music and ensembles, 100–3, 134, 144–45
   childhood perspectives, documenting, 20–21
   coherence and continuity in, 27–28
   on conscientiousness and artistry, 68–69, 72, 140
   cross-disciplinary perspectives on dimensions of, 30–33, 31*t*
   on dispositional musicality, 64–65
   on disruption and renewal of musical plans, 88–107, 144–48
   on embodiment, 65–67
   on extraversion and performance, 69–71, 138–39, 140
   on grandparents, 48–50, 133–34
   on instrument choice and identity, 75–78, 84, 99–100
   memories of musical experiences in, 27–28, 35–38
   memory, truth, and values in, 23–24
   memory and emotion in, 22–23
   on musical kinship, 78–83, 133–35
   musical selves conceptualized in, 61–62
   on music at home, 38–40
   on music in church, 41–42
   on music in family car, 42–43
   on music in neighborhoods and societal contexts, 52–54
   on neuroticism and vulnerability of emotional expression, 72–75, 140
   on openness to experience, 71–72, 73, 74, 140
   on parents, 43–48, 52, 133
   on performing together, kinship and, 81–83
   reconstructing and remembering, 21–24
   on siblings, 50–52, 134
   teaching narratives and generativity, 107–10

music making, by children, 2–3, 141
   adults' encounters with, 29–30
   enchantment and, 117
   in family culture, 38
   family members documenting, 45
   as improvisational, 131
   in intimate, communal settings, 14
   with mothers, 45
   music as transitional object and, 14
   on playgrounds, 11–12
   privacy in, 136
   ritual in, 38–39, 40
   spontaneous, 8, 37, 39–40, 135–36
music teaching, generativity and, 107–10
mutuality, 2, 38, 44, 50, 57, 82, 114, 115, 133–35, 151
Myers-Briggs personality traits, 69
My Lord, What a Morning (Anderson), 79

Nachmanovitch, Stephen, 131
Nadeau, ReNee, 100–1
National Association for Music Education (NAfME), 96
New Horizon band programs, 81
"New World Symphony," 82
New York City Ballet, 80
Nutcracker, The, 80
Nutcracker Suite, The, 9

Ondaatje, Michael, 129
opera, for infants, 117–27, 119*f*, 156–57

Pachelbel, Johann, 109
parents
   in childhood musical experiences, 43–48, 52, 57
   singing, 45–47, 57, 107, 133, 135, 141
   as teachers, 156–57
Parents Use of Music with Infants Study, 54
Paterson, Lliam, 119–21, 122, 124
"Pathétique Sonata," 13
Paul, Les, 22–23
Pazant, Alvin, 80
Pazant, Ed, 80
periodicity, 6
Perlman, Itzhak, 65, 77
Piaget, Jean, 132–33

Pieces of Light (Ferneyhough), 23–24
Pigrum, D., 44
Pilkauskas, N., 48
postpartum depression, 12–13
Preludio y Merengue, 102–3
Puente, Tito, 39–40

Rasmussen, A. S., 22, 23, 24
Recchia, Susan, 118
reconstructing, remembering and, 21–24
remembering, reconstructing and, 21–24
resilience, 73, 146
road trips, 87–88
Rodgers and Hammerstein, 136

Schoenberg, Arnold, 81–82
Scottish Opera, 117–18
SDASA Chorale, 57–58, 149
self-regulation, 7–8
SEM. *See* strong experiences with music
Shafer, R. Murray, 3
Sheehan Campbell, Patricia, 2
siblings, in childhood musical
    experiences, 50–52, 134
Siegel, Daniel, 22
Simunye concert, 57–58, 149
Sinatra, Frank, 52
singing, 9–10, 13–14, 37–38, 84
    with family members, 43
    intimacy and, 136
    in narratives of disruption and renewal,
        92, 93, 94, 95, 96–98
    by parents, 45–47, 57, 107, 133, 135, 141
    spontaneous, 135–36
"16 Candles," 69–70
social action, developmental pathways
    of, 143*t*
social actors, 61–62, 66, 67, 70,
    138, 141–42
Sole, M., 13
"Song for Mama, A," 97
"Sospan Fach," 53
sound groups, 10–13, 38–43, 133–35, 142
Sound of Music, The, 64–65
stability, change and, 137–44
Stern, D. N., 5, 126

"Stop in the Name of Love," 70
Stravinsky, Igor, 101
strong experiences with music (SEM), 23
Supremes, the, 70
Suzuki Method, 77, 81, 103–4, 106
"Sweet Georgia Brown," 42–43
symbiosis, 40, 57–58
Symphony No. 7 (Dvořák), 51
synchronicity, 114, 145, 157–58
synchrony, 7–8, 12–13

Tagore, Rabindranath, 146–47
Tchaikovsky, Pyotr Ilyich, 9, 13, 80
teaching, in responsive
    partnership, 146–48
Theodorakis, Mikis, 1–2
"This Land Is Your Land," 61
transcendence, 73
transitional object, music as, 13–
    14, 44, 57
transitional practices, 44
trauma, 87–88, 92, 97, 144, 146, 157
Trehub, S. E., 63
Turino, T., 57

Ungar, 146

Vandross, Luther, 96–97
Van Manen, M., 136
Verdi, Giuseppe, 74
Verklärte Nacht, 81–82

Weber, Carl Maria von, 101
"What a Wonderful World," 136–37
Wiggins, 73
Williams, Vaughan, 97–98
Wilson, Graeme, 131
Wilson, Nancy, 132
Winnecott, D. W., 13–14
Wittgenstein, Ludwig, 112
wonder, discovery and, 151–53

Yeats, W. B., 7
Yi, Tammy, 151
"You Are the Woman That I Always
    Dreamed Of," 61

The manufacturer's authorised representative in the EU for product safety is Oxford
University Press España S.A. of El Parque Empresarial San Fernando de Henares,
Avenida de Castilla, 2 – 28830 Madrid (www.oup.es/en or product.safety@oup.com).
OUP España S.A. also acts as importer into Spain of products made by the manufacturer.

Printed in the USA/Agawam, MA
March 21, 2025

884675.007